Trigger Point Therapy

for

Lower Back and Gluteal Pain

(Second Edition)

Valerie DeLaune, LAc

INSTITUTE OF
TRIGGER POINT
STUDIES
TRIGGERPOINTRELIEF.COM

ISBN 13: 978-0-9968553-2-7

First Edition, 2012
Second Edition, 2013

Disclaimer:
The following information is intended for general information purposes only. Individuals should always see their health care provider before administering any suggestions made in this book. Any application of the material set forth in the following pages is at the reader's discretion and is his or her sole responsibility.

This book is intended as a quick-reference only for the major muscles that may harbor trigger points that refer pain to the lower back and gluteal areas. It is not intended as a comprehensive therapy guide for other areas of the body. If you are unable to relieve all of your pain with the techniques found in this book, you may wish to consult one of the resources found at the end of this book in order to treat other pertinent muscles.

Table of Contents

Acknowledgements / About the Author 1

Chapter 1: Locating and Treating Trigger Points: General Guidelines 3

Chapter 2: Trigger Point Location Guide 9

Chapter 3: Paraspinals 12

Chapter 4: Iliopsoas 23

Chapter 5: Abdominals 29

Chapter 6: Quadratus Lumborum 38

Chapter 7: Gluteus Medius 45

Chapter 8: Gluteus Minimus 50

Chapter 9: Gluteus Maximus 57

Chapter 10: Piriformis 61

Chapter 11: Hamstrings 67

Chapter 12: Pelvic Floor 72

Appendix A: Perpetuating Factors 76

Appendix B: What Are Trigger Points? 96

Other Books by the Author 102

Acknowledgements

This book would not have been possible without the lifeworks of Dr. Janet Travell and Dr. David G. Simons, who worked endlessly to research trigger points, document referral patterns and other symptoms, and bring all of that information to medical practitioners and the general public. Together Doctors Travell and Simons produced a comprehensive two-volume text on the causes and treatment of trigger points, written for physicians. This text is a condensation of those volumes, written for the general public, and for practitioners who don't need the in-depth knowledge to perform trigger point injections.

Dr. Janet Travell and Dr. David G. Simons

Dr. Travell pioneered and researched new pain treatments, including trigger point injections. In her private practice, she began treating Senator John F. Kennedy, who at the time was using crutches due to crippling back pain and was almost unable to walk down just a few stairs. It had become important for presidential candidates to appear physically fit, because of television. Being on crutches probably would have cost President Kennedy the election. Dr. Travell became the first female White House physician, and after President Kennedy died, she stayed on to treat President Johnson. She resigned a year and a half later to return to her passions: teaching, lecturing, and writing about chronic myofascial pain. She continued to work into her nineties and died at the age of ninety-five on August 1, 1997.

Dr. Simons met Dr. Travell when she lectured at the School of Aerospace Medicine at Brooks Air Force Base in Texas in the 1960s. He soon teamed up with Dr. Travell and began researching the international literature for any references to the treatment of pain. There were a few others out there who were also discovering trigger points but using different terminology. He studied and documented the physiology of trigger points in both laboratory and clinical settings and tried to find scientific explanations for trigger points. He continued to research the physiology of trigger points, update the trigger point volumes he coauthored with Dr. Travell, and review trigger point research articles until his death at the age of 88 on April 5, 2010.

I am also profoundly grateful to my neuromuscular therapy instructor, Jeanne Aland, who taught me basics about trigger points, and introduced me to the books written by Doctors Travell and Simons. I was told Jeanne passed on a few years ago.

All three are well-missed. Those familiar with trigger points are extremely grateful for their hard work and dedication. Their work lives on through the hundreds of thousands of patients who have gotten relief because of their research and willingness to train others.

Other Thanks

Many additional researchers have contributed to the study of trigger points, and many doctors and other practitioners have taken the time to learn about trigger points and give that information to their patients. I would like to acknowledge all of them for their role in alleviating pain by making this important information available. In particular I would like to thank Dr. Juhani Partanen, who kindly explained the "Muscle Spindle" hypothesis to me in lay terms, and also took the time to review "Appendix B -- What Are Trigger Points" to make sure I had translated scientific language correctly into easier-to-understand terms.

My Background

I attended massage school in 1989 and learned Swedish massage. I learned to give a very good general massage, but I didn't feel equipped to treat chronic pain. I was very intrigued by a description of a continuing education certificate course; it was called *neuromuscular therapy,* which combines *myofascial release* (a type of deep tissue massage) with treating trigger points. I attended the class in 1991, taught by Jeanne Aland at Heartwood Institute, and it completely changed my approach to treating patients. Once I learned about referral patterns, I was able to consistently resolve chronic pain problems.

Over my years of treating thousands of patients, I have added my own observations to those of Doctors Travell and Simons, and developed a variety of self-help techniques, which are included in my books.

In 1999, I received my master's degree in acupuncture. Since then I've been writing trigger point books and articles, teaching trigger point continuing education classes to health care providers, and specializing in treating pain syndromes by combining dry-needling of trigger points with Traditional Chinese Medicine diagnosis and treatment.

Valerie DeLaune, LAc

Chapter 1: Locating and Treating Trigger Points: General Guidelines

Where to Start?

Chapter 2 contains the *Trigger Point Location Guide;* this will help you figure out which muscles in this book may harbor trigger points that might be causing your symptoms. Locate your pain or other symptoms for each area, and then refer to the chapters listed.

Each muscle chapter has drawings that show the most common pain referral areas for each trigger point. The more solid black or white area indicates the primary area of referral, which is almost always present, and the lighter stippled area shows the most likely secondary areas of referral, which may or may not be present. Keep in mind that the referral patterns only show the most *common* referral patterns; your referral pattern may be somewhat different or even completely different. You may also have overlapping referral patterns from trigger points in multiple muscles. These areas may be more extensive than the patterns common for individual muscles, and pain may be more intense. For this reason, over time, be sure to search for trigger points in all the muscles that refer pain to that area.

Each muscle chapter contains an anatomical drawing of the muscle or muscles covered in that chapter, with "X"'s showing some of the most common locations of trigger points. *There may be additional trigger points or they may be in different places, so search the entire muscle.* Keep in mind that for some muscles, the "X" may just be an *example* of a trigger point location and its associated referral pattern, but they may occur at any level; for example, trigger points in the *paraspinal* muscles.

Each muscle chapter also includes lists of common symptoms and factors that may cause or perpetuate trigger points. Again, these are only the most common; you may experience different symptoms, and your causes and perpetuating factors may be different. If you think you might have trigger points in a certain muscle but don't see any perpetuating factors that apply to you, try to imagine whether anything in your life is similar to something on the list that could be causing the same type of stress on the muscle.

Once you've determined which two muscles most closely fit your pain referral pattern and symptoms, start doing the self-help pressure and stretching, and eliminate the applicable perpetuating factors. Over the next several weeks, search for trigger points in additional muscles, and add those into your treatment regime as needed. As you start to feel better, you'll develop a clearer picture of which trigger points are causing your pain, and which perpetuating factors are reactivating your trigger points.

Other Things to Consider...

When you apply pressure to the trigger point, you can often reproduce the referred pain or other symptoms, but being unable to reproduce the referred pain or other symptoms by applying pressure does *not* rule out involvement of that specific trigger point. Try treating the trigger points that could be causing the problem anyway, and if you improve, even temporarily, assume that one of the trigger points you worked on is indeed at least part of the problem. For this reason, don't work on all the possible trigger points in one session, since you won't know which trigger point treated actually gave you relief.

Be aware that a *primary*, or *key*, trigger point can cause a *satellite* trigger point to develop in a different muscle. The satellite trigger point may have formed for one of these reasons: it lies within the referral zone of the primary trigger point, or it's in a muscle that is either substituting for, or is countering tension for the muscle that contains the primary trigger point. When doing self-treatments, be aware that if some of your trigger points are satellite trigger points, you won't get lasting relief until the primary trigger points have been treated. This is why it is important to work in the direction of referral (see "Do's" below).

You also need to be aware that central sensitization (explained in Appendix B) can cause the referral pattern to deviate from the most common pattern found in each muscle chapter. It may also cause trigger points in several muscles within a region to refer pain to the same area, making it more difficult to determine trigger point locations. This means you can't absolutely rule out the role of a potential trigger point based *only* on consideration of common referral patterns, since other factors may cause you to have an *uncommon* referral pattern. The more intense the earlier pain, the more intense the emotions associated with it, and the longer pain has lasted, the more likely central sensitization will cause deviation from the most common referral patterns.

A small percentage of people will get worse before they get better, mostly in complex cases. Or the pain may move around, or you may have the perception that the pain moved around only because the most painful areas have improved and now you are noticing the next most painful area more. I've only had a few cases where I wasn't able to help patients, because they were so frustrated after receiving little or no help from professional after professional that they only allowed me to treat them a few times before giving up, *even if they had improved*. If you get a little worse before you get better, you may be inclined to give up in the initial stages of treatment. I encourage you to give any treatment you try some amount of time before you decide it isn't working, even if your condition initially gets worse.

General Guidelines for Applying Self-Pressure

DON'Ts:

- **Do not apply pressure over varicose veins, open wounds, infections, herniated/bulging disks, areas of phlebitis/thrombophlebitis, or where clots are present or could be present. If you are pregnant, do not apply pressure on your legs.**

- **Most importantly: *Don't overdo the self-help techniques!*** Many people think that if some feels great, more will be even better, but you can actually make yourself worse by not following the guidelines. Expect gradual improvement, though you may improve most quickly during the initial weeks of therapy.

DO's:

- **Use a tennis ball, racquetball, golf ball, dog play ball, or baseball, or use your elbow or hand if instructed for particular muscles.** For balls, use the weight of your body to give you the pressure; don't press your back or limb onto the balls. The muscle you are working on should be as passive as possible. Use one ball at a time on your back, not one on each side.

- **Apply pressure for a minimum of eight seconds, and a maximum of one minute;** less than eight seconds may activate trigger points, and more than a minute will cut off the circulation for too long and make it worse. Time yourself first to be sure you are actually counting seconds at the correct speed.

- **It should be somewhat uncomfortable, or "hurt good," but it should not be so painful that you are either tensing up or holding your breath. If it is too painful, use a smaller or softer ball, or move to a softer surface (like a bed, or pad your surface with a pillow or blanket).** If it does *not* hurt at all, keep looking for tender spots, or try moving to a harder surface. If it's too tender to lie on, try putting a ball in a long sock and leaning against the wall. I only recommend using the wall if you cannot lie on the ball, since you are then using the very muscles you are trying to work on. You may need to use a combination of surfaces depending on the tenderness of different areas. Over time, as sensitivity decreases, you may need to change ball dimensions and/or hardness, or move to a harder surface.

- **Search the *entire* muscle for tender points, particularly the points of maximum tenderness.** Use the pictures to make sure you are getting the entire muscle and not just the worst spot. Many times a tendon attachment will hurt because the tight muscle is pulling on it, but if you don't treat the bulk of the muscle, it will keep pulling on the attachment.

- **Be sure to work on both sides of the body to keep the muscles balanced, but spend more time on the areas that need it more.** Except for very new one-sided injuries, the same muscle on the opposite side will almost always be tender with pressure, even if it has not yet started causing symptoms. If you loosen one side but not the other, it can lead to additional problems. Sometimes problems with the muscles on the opposite side are actually causing the symptoms, so it is always worth working on both sides.

- **Work in the direction of referral.** For example, if your gluteal muscles hurt and the pain is being referred from trigger points in the *quadratus lumborum* muscle in the lumbar area, work on the lumbar area first, then the gluteal area.

- If you have limited time, **do one area thoroughly rather than rushing through many areas.** You are more likely to aggravate trigger points rather than inactivate them if you rush.

- **Do stretches *after* the trigger point work.** If you only have time to do one thing, do the ball/pressure work and skip the stretches.

- **Most people should work on their muscles one time per day initially.** If you have an appointment with your therapist, do not do your self-help the same day. If you are sore from your therapy appointment or your self-help, skip a day. If you are sore for more than one day or your symptoms get worse, it is likely that either the pressure was too hard or you held points for too long. Review these guidelines if that is the case. Tell your therapist if you are sore from their work. This is *not* a case of where if some is great, more is better.

    Pick a time when you will remember to do your self-help, i.e., when you wake up, when you watch television, or when you go to bed, and keep your balls by the bed (*but do not fall asleep on a ball!*).

    After a few weeks, you may wish to increase your self-help to twice per day, as long as you are not getting sore. If a particular activity bothers you, you may wish to do the self-help before and after the activity. If you start getting sore or your symptoms get worse, decrease your self-help frequency.

    Treat your trigger points for as long as they are sensitive, even if active symptoms have disappeared. If trigger points are still tender, they are *latent*, and could easily be reactivated. Most likely you will start forgetting as symptoms disappear; however, the most important thing you will have learned is what to do if your symptoms return.

- **If you have questions or your symptoms get worse, or you are sore for more than one day, stop the self-help until you have had a chance to consult with your therapist.** They should be able to help you figure out any problems.

- **Take your balls on trips with you,** since travel frequently aggravates trigger points. You may even wish to keep some balls at work.

General Guidelines for Stretches and Conditioning

It is very important to distinguish the difference between *stretching* and *conditioning* exercises. *Stretching* means you gently lengthen the muscle fibers. *Conditioning* means you are trying to strengthen the muscle. Doctors Travell and Simons found that *active* trigger points benefited from stretching, but were usually aggravated by conditioning exercises. Once trigger points have been *inactivated*, conditioning is beneficial. Make sure your physical therapist or physiotherapist is familiar with trigger points, and begins your therapy with stretching exercises.

Usually two weeks of trigger point self-help treatment will be sufficient before adding in conditioning exercises, but if your trigger points are still very irritable, you will need to wait until your symptoms improve. Meanwhile, learn the stretches in this book. If you are not sure whether an assigned activity is a stretch or conditioning, ask your practitioner. I will not cover guidelines for conditioning exercises in depth here, since your physical therapist or physiotherapist will prescribe them.

DON'Ts:

- **Don't bounce on stretches, and avoid stretching when your muscles are tired or cold.**

- **Don't do a conditioning exercise just because it worked for someone else.** Doctors Travell and Simons said "Exercise should be regarded as a prescription, much as one prescribes medication. Like a drug, there is a right kind, dose, and timing of exercise." Often a friend will recommend an exercise that worked for them, but you are a different person with a different set of symptoms, and you should no more do their assigned exercises than you would take their prescribed medications. Be sure to tell your therapist all of the activities and exercises/stretches you are doing, because one of these can be contributing to your trigger point activation.

- **Don't keep doing an exercise or stretch that is aggravating your symptoms.** Check with your therapist to determine why it is bothering you and to find out how to proceed.

DO's:

- **Stretch slowly, and only to the point of just getting a gentle stretch; *don't force it.*** If you stretch the muscles too hard or too fast, you can aggravate trigger points.

- **Hold your stretch for 30 to 60 seconds.** There will be little benefit after 30 seconds, but it will not hurt you to stretch for longer either. You may repeat the stretch after releasing and breathing.

- **For any type of repetitive exercise, breathe and rest between each cycle of the exercise.**

- **If you are sore for more than one day** from exercises or stretches, reduce the number of repetitions and try again after the soreness has disappeared. If you are still sore for two days after the exercise or stretch, it needs to be changed.

General Guidelines for Muscle Care

These are some general suggestions for taking care of your muscles; each muscle chapter will have specific suggestions.

DON'Ts:

- Never put the maximum load on a muscle -- it is too easy to strain it.

- Don't lift something too heavy -- ask for help.

- Don't keep muscles in positions of sustained contractions, where you are holding them tense or in sustained use. In order to increase blood flow and bring oxygen and nutrients to the muscles, they need to alternately constrict and relax.

- Don't sit for too long in one position.

- Don't expose your muscles to cold drafts.

DO's:

- After treatments, gently use the muscle in a normal way that uses its full range-of-motion, but avoid strenuous activities immediately afterward or until the trigger points aren't so easily aggravated, whichever is longer.

- Vary your activities so you are not doing any one thing for too long. Rest and take breaks frequently from any given activity.

- Lift with your knees bent and your back straight, with the object close to your chest.

- Notice where you hold tension and practice relaxing those areas.

- Swimming is generally a good exercise, and bicycling is easier on the body than running, but in both cases, take care to avoid straining the trapezius and neck muscles. A recumbent, stationary, or other bike that allows you to sit more upright is preferable.

- When starting an exercise program, *underestimate* what you will be able to do. Gradually add increments in duration, rate, and effort, and in amounts that will not cause you to be sore or activate trigger points.

- Warm-up adequately for sports activities.

- If you are working with a practitioner, they should be able to help you prioritize what needs to be done in order of most importance. If your practitioner is giving you too many things to do at once, be sure to tell them that you are overwhelmed and need to set priorities. Giving a patient too many assignments is all too easy for a practitioner to do, especially when they are first out of school and brimming with many useful ideas and suggestions.

Be sure to return to this chapter often to review the guidelines to ensure you are treating the muscles properly, particularly if something is not working for you, or trigger points are getting aggravated instead of inactivated. Chances are you have forgotten to follow these guidelines.

Be sure to set realistic goals. Focus on a few muscles at a time unless there is a reason that you need to work on several together. Setting unrealistic goals can discourage you, and cause you to give up. It's better to pick just a few things and do them well rather than rush through too many self-help techniques or suggestions and do them poorly. You probably won't be able to apply pressure on five different muscles and stretch them, get orthotics and replace bad shoes, change your diet, and start walking every day all in the first week. Pace yourself so that this is an enjoyable process, and work on the perpetuating factors over time.

Chapter 2: Trigger Point Location Guide

To figure out which muscles to work on first, look at the trigger point location guides and refer to the chapters listed for each. Examine the photos of referral patterns in each chapter and try to find those that most closely match your pain pattern, and read the list of symptoms for each muscle. Refer to chapter 1 for additional instructions on locating and treating trigger points, and general guidelines for applying pressure, stretching, and general muscle care.

1. Paraspinals (3)
   Iliopsoas (4)
   Rectus abdominis (5)
   Gluteus medius (7)
   Iliolumbar ligament (6)

2. Pelvic floor (12)
   Gluteus medius (7)
   Quadratus lumborum (6)
   Gluteus maximus (9)
   Multifidi (3)
   Rectus abdominis (5)

3. Gluteus medius (7)
   Quadratus lumborum (6)
   Gluteus maximus (9)
   Paraspinals (3)
   Semitendinosus / Semimembranosus (11)
   Iliolumbar ligament (6)
   Piriformis (10)
   Gluteus minimus (8)
   Rectus abdominis (5)
   Pelvic floor (12)

Muscle chapters for all of the remaining areas of the body can be found in *Pain Relief with Trigger Point Self-Help.* Please see the end of this book for more information.

Blank Body Chart

You may wish to make copies of the following blank body chart and draw your symptom pattern on one of them with a colored marker. Then you can compare your pattern with the pain referral pictures in chapters 3 through 12. Out to the side of each painful area, note your pain intensity on a scale of 1 to 10 and the percent of time you feel pain in that area—for example, 6.5/80%. (If you are unable to print from your device, go to http://triggerpointrelief.com/pain_guides.html for a copy you can print off.)

I recommend that you fill out a body chart at least a couple of times per week. Date them so that you'll be able to keep them in order. This chronological record will come in handy in several ways. It will:

- make it easier for you to discern which patterns fit your pain referral most closely;
- help you recognize the factors that cause and perpetuate your symptoms by matching fluctuations in the level and frequency of your symptoms;
- allow you to track your progress (or lack thereof) and provide a historical record of any injuries.

As your condition improves, you may forget how intense your symptoms were originally, and you may think you're not getting any better. You'll be able to see that you are improving, even if you have an occasional setback. One thing to note, however, is that not everyone can accurately draw their pain location, due in part to lack of familiarity with anatomy, so take that possibility into consideration and check muscles with adjacent referral patterns just in case your drawing is inaccurate.

Chapter 3: Paraspinals

(Iliocostalis Lumborum, Iliocostalis Thoracis,
Longissimus Thoracis, Multifidi)

Part of this muscle group runs the entire length of the spine, and some of the muscles run most of the length of the spine. Yet others (the *multifidi*) are small muscles that attach one vertebra to the next. These are the muscles that allow you to bend and twist.

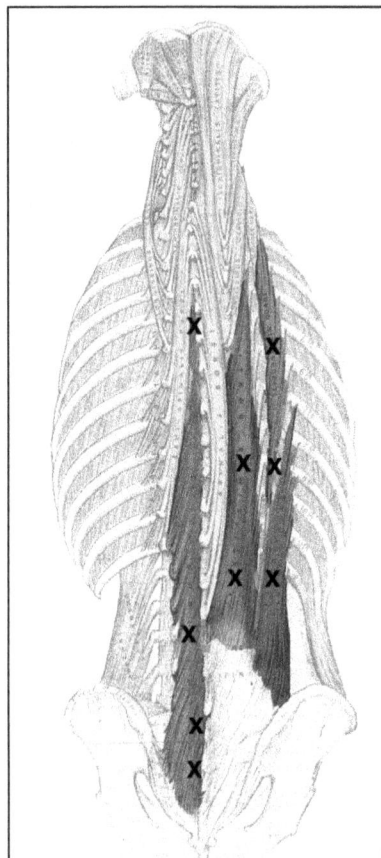

Back view of trunk

Common Symptoms

- See the pictures for all the pain referral patterns. These pictures show common trigger points, *but trigger points can develop at any level and cause similar referral patterns at any level*. Please note that in many cases pain can refer to the front side of the body, causing you to think you are having organ problems, particularly in the area of the heart. Trigger points in these muscles are an often overlooked cause of buttocks pain.
- deep, aching pain that feels like it is in the spine
- pain may increase with coughing or straining to have a bowel movement
- restricted range-of-motion or restricted rotation of the trunk, possibly severe
- possibly difficulty climbing stairs or getting out of a chair
- possibly nausea, belching, and gastrointestinal pain and cramping

- entrapment of spinal nerves cause increased or decreased sensitivity and/or uncomfortable sensations on the skin of the back
- stiffness in the spine, mostly from the *longissimus thoracis*

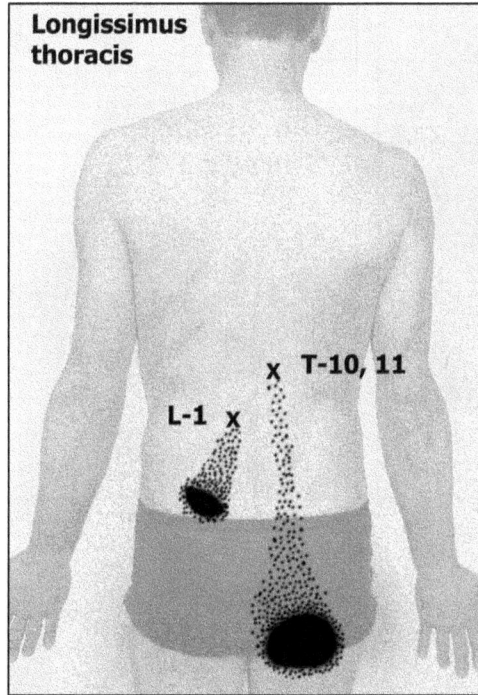

Iliocostalis lumborum

Longissimus thoracis

T-10, 11

L-1

Sample referral patterns, but all of these can occur at any level of the back.

Iliocostalis thoracis T-6

Back referral pattern

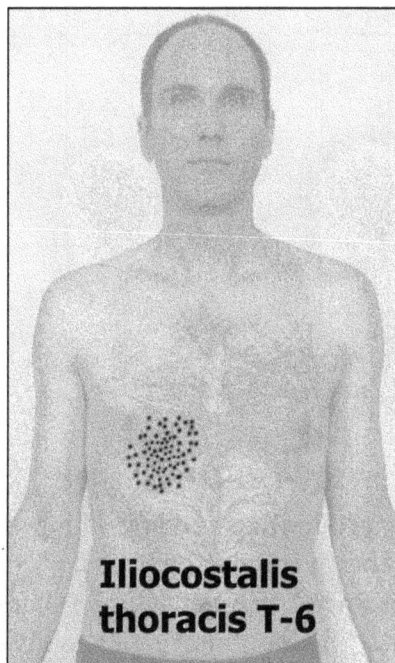

Iliocostalis thoracis T-6

Front referral pattern

Iliocostalis thoracis T-11

Iliocostalis thoracis T-11

Sample referral patterns, but all of these can occur at any level of the back.

Back referral pattern

Front referral pattern

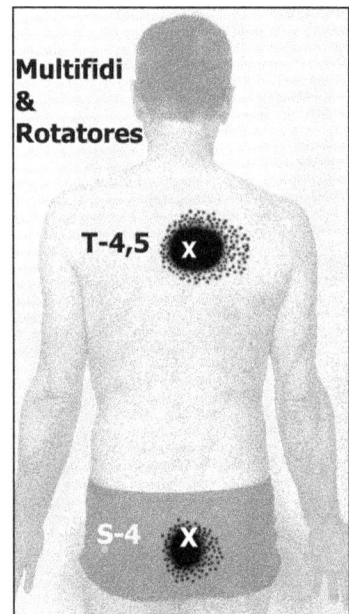

Multifidi

Multifidi

Multifidi & Rotatores

L-2

X S-1

L-2

S-1

T-4,5 X

S-4 X

Back referral pattern

Front referral pattern

Causes and Perpetuation of Trigger Points

- a sudden overload, often when bending, lifting, and twisting at the same time (people frequently tell me they were moving boxes)
- catching yourself from falling, such as when slipping on ice
- sitting for long periods without moving, in as little as hour or less for some people
- sitting on a wallet in your back pocket
- bending over while gardening

- injury is more likely when the muscles are chilled or fatigued
- car accidents, especially a whiplash injury
- mattresses that are too old or too soft, or sleeping next to someone who is heavier and trying to avoid rolling into them
- a tight belt or bra strap
- trigger points in the *latissimus dorsi* (a muscle covering the back and sides of the trunk)
- head-forward posture
- one leg anatomically shorter than the other (this does *not* refer to the "short leg" terminology chiropractors often use to describe the effect of vertebrae being out-of-alignment), or an unequal hemipelvis size (either the right or left half of the pelvis)

This is a list of perpetuating factors specific only to trigger points in <u>these</u> *muscles. For a full list of perpetuating factors that can cause and perpetuate trigger points anywhere in the body and which also apply to these muscles, please see "Appendix A" (found at the end of this book), since some may need to be addressed for lasting pain relief*

Helpful Hints
- Don't keep a wallet in a back pocket, since it will tilt your pelvis and spine when sitting.
- Modify or replace your mis-fitting furniture. Your knees should fit under your desk, and the chair needs to be close enough that you can lean against your backrest. Your elbows should rest on either your work surface or armrests at the same height. Your elbows and forearms should rest evenly on the armrests. Your computer screen should be directly in front of you, and the copy attached to the side of the screen, so that you may look directly forward as much as possible. Take frequent breaks.
- Get a headset or speaker for your phone, or hold the phone with one hand. Shoulder rests are not adequate.
- If you must bend over plans or reading materials (such as a draftsman, engineer, or architect), a tilted work surface will alleviate the mechanical stress to a point, but be sure to take frequent breaks.
- Lift properly by bending your knees rather than your back, and hold objects close to your body.
- Wear bras that fit properly. If you see elastic marks on your skin after you take your bra off, the straps are too tight. Jogging bras work great for medium or small-breasted women. Have the salesperson help you find a bra that fits properly -- many of them really know their products.
- If you are gardening, straighten up frequently, and stand and stretch periodically.
- Be sure to slide into the center of your car seat. Some bucket seats curve up on each side, and if you are not in the center, your pelvis is tilted.
- Buy a firm mattress, and replace it every five to seven years. You can put plywood between the box springs and mattress to make it firmer.
- If you have difficulty getting up, roll over onto your hands and knees and crawl to where you can grab onto something and pull yourself up.
- When standing up from a chair, slide your butt to the front of the chair, turn your entire body a little sideways, put one foot under the front edge of the chair, then stand with

your torso erect so that your thighs take the load. You can use your hands to assist you if necessary. Sit down in the opposite sequence.

- When climbing stairs or a ladder, rotate your entire body 45-degrees and keep your back straight.
- Restoration of proper posture, especially head positioning, is critical to treating trigger points since head-forward posture can both cause and perpetuate **trigger points**. Head-forward posture can be aggravated while sitting in a car, at a desk, in front of a computer, or while eating dinner or watching TV. Using a good lumbar support everywhere you sit will help correct poor sitting posture.   See the exercise below in the "Self-Help Techniques" section for postural re-training.

Poor posture   *Good Posture*

- If you have a body asymmetry or an anatomically shorter leg, see a specialist to get compensating lifts or pads.

Self-Help Techniques

Applying Pressure

Paraspinal Pressure: The shading on the picture marks the area you will want to work on.

Lie face-up on a firm bed or the floor, with your knees bent. Using a tennis ball or racquet ball, start at the shoulder, about one inch out to the side of the spine, and hold pressure for eight seconds to one minute per spot. Shift a small amount to the next spot further down the back by using your legs to move your body over the ball, and continue to hold pressure on each spot. Continue working down all the way to the top of the pelvis in order to treat both the *trapezius* and the *paraspinal* muscles. You may want to repeat this on a second line further out from the spine, especially if you have a wide back or if you have tender points further out. *Do not do this directly on the spine!* I recommend using one ball at a time, rather than using a ball on each side at the same time. By performing this technique lying down, as opposed to standing and leaning into the wall, you keep the muscles as passive as possible, so that you are not using them to hold you upright while you are applying pressure.

If you are at work and unable to lie on the floor, I recommend using a Backnobber® from Pressure Positive Company (see below).

Longissimus thoracis pressure: To work on the *longissimus thoracis*, which is very close to the spine, you will need to lie on a hard floor and use a golf ball. Place the golf ball *in between* your spine and the muscle (not *on* the spine—see photo), and then move your body just a little *away* from the side you are working on. This presses on the muscles at a 45° angle, the only really effective way to get this muscle. Do this from the bottom of the neck, down to the top of the pelvis. As a trigger point therapist, I perform this treatment by standing on the opposite side and leaning across, pressing the muscle out at a 45° angle.

Demonstrating location of muscle and direction to press out against golf ball

Lay on a golf ball to perform this self-help technique

Multifidi pressure: To treat the *multifidi* (the little muscles that attach one vertebra to the next), you will need the assistance of another person, as even a golf ball is too large. They will need a tool, such as a rubber-tipped wooden dowel (available at a massage supply store), or an eraser that is rounded off. Working next to the spinous process (the pointy part of the vertebra), massage in the groove next to it. Your assistant may be able to use their thumb, but a gadget works better and is easier on the person administering the treatment.

Backnobber®: If you are at work and unable to lie on the floor, I recommend using a Backnobber® from Pressure Positive Company to apply pressure to the *paraspinal* muscles. Note how both hands are pulling the Backnobber® away from the body in the direction the arrows are pointing, rather than pressing it into the front of the trunk to lever pressure onto the back.

Posterior Neck Pressure: I find it is best to treat the *paraspinal* muscles first and the *posterior neck* muscles second.

The shading in the picture marks the area to work on. You may work along the base of the skull and down the back of the neck. Try to get all the way to the base of the neck where it intersects the top of the shoulder, in order to work on the entire *splenius cervicis* muscle.

To treat the back of your neck, use a golf ball and lie face-up with your hands behind your neck. One palm should be squarely over the other palm, with the golf ball in the center of your top palm, and *not* where the fingers join the palm.

Keep your head relaxed throughout the self-treatment. To apply pressure, rotate your head toward the ball. Be sure to work on the muscles to the *side* of the spine—don't put the ball directly *on* the spine. To move the ball, roll your head away from the side you are working on, move the ball a small amount, and then rotate your head back toward the side you are working on. If you want more pressure, rotate your head toward the side you are working on even more; rotate your head less if you want less pressure. *Do not raise your head to move the ball.* This will cause additional stress on the muscles, so be sure to move the ball by *rotating* your head away from it.

Stretches

In-Bathtub Stretch: With your head hanging forward, lean forward and reach your hands down toward your toes, until you are feeling a gentle stretch. Relax and then repeat, moving your hands further down each time, but only as far down as you can feel a gentle stretch. Do this in a hot bath if you can. [**Note**: If you have trigger points in the *iliopsoas* muscle, even if they are latent, this stretch can cause a reactive cramp. You may need to work on and stretch the *iliopsoas* first; see chapter 4.]

Low Back Stretching Exercise: Lying on your back, with your hands clasped *behind* one knee, gently bring that knee toward your chest until you are just feeling the stretch. Repeat with the opposite knee, and then both legs at the same time.

Posterior Neck Stretch: You may do this stretch under a hot shower and, if possible, seated on a stool. Lock your fingers behind your head and pull your head gently forward. Turn your head to one side at a 45° angle and gently pull your head in that direction. Place one hand on the top of your head and gently pull your head down to that side. Repeat on the opposite side.

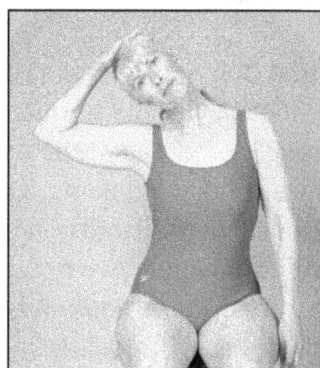

Exercises

Postural Re-training: Postural exercises can help eliminate head-forward posture. To learn proper posture and correct a head-forward position, stand with your feet about four inches apart, with your arms at your sides and thumbs pointing forward. Tighten your buttocks to stabilize your lower back, then, while inhaling, rotate your arms and shoulders out and back by rotating your thumbs backward, and squeeze the shoulder blades together in the back. Keep holding this position while dropping your shoulders down and exhaling. Move your head back to bring your ears in line with your shoulders and hold this position for about six seconds while breathing normally.

When moving your head, don't move your nose up or down, or open your mouth. Relax, but then try to maintain good posture once you release the pose. If holding this position feels uncomfortable or "stiff," try shifting your body weight from your heels to the balls of your feet, which causes your head to move backward over your shoulders. This exercise should be repeated frequently during the day in order to retrain yourself in good postural techniques, at least every one to two hours. It is better to do one repetition six or more times per day than to do six repetitions in a row.

Also See:

* Iliopsoas (chapter 4)
* Quadratus lumborum (chapter 6)

You may also need to search for trigger points in the *serratus posterior superior*, *serratus posterior inferior*, and *latissimus dorsi*, since trigger points in those muscles can either cause similar pain referral patterns or may affect or be affected by *paraspinal* trigger points in some way.

Since trigger points in these muscles don't directly cause lower back and gluteal pain, they are not addressed in this book. If you can't relieve your pain with the self-help techniques in this book after six to eight weeks, you may wish to consider whether you need to treat trigger points in these additional muscles, or if you still have perpetuating factors to resolve. Go to the end of this book for other books by the author that provide self-treatment techniques of muscles not covered in this book.

Differential Diagnosis: If you are experiencing pain in the spine, you will need to see a health care provider to rule out herniated discs, spinal stenosis (narrowing of the hole the spinal cord goes through, or of one of the holes the nerves go out through), infections, tumors, cancer, or other more serious problems. Other diagnoses that should be considered are fibromyalgia, organ disease, osteoarthritis, fat lobules, strain of spinal ligaments, retrocecal appendicitis, a dissecting aortic aneurysm or saddle thrombus, kidney stones, torsion of the kidney, pelvic inflammatory disease, endometriosis, ankylosing spondylitis, Paget's disease, leukemia, Hodgkin's disease, prostatitis and seminal vesiculitis, or sacroiliitis. A finding of osteoarthritis in itself may not account for the pain felt, since you can have pain without degenerative changes to the spine, and you can have degenerative changes without pain. Lumbar zygapophysial (facet) joints may refer pain in the same pattern as multifidi muscles.

Vertebrae may be out of alignment and need to be adjusted by a chiropractor or osteopathic physician. Combining acupuncture or massage with adjustments is more helpful, since tight muscles will keep pulling vertebra out of alignment.

Chapter 4: Iliopsoas

Front View of Abdomen and Thigh

Common Symptoms

- the upper part of the muscle (the ***psoas***) attaches to the front sides of T-12 and the lumbar vertebrae, and primarily refers pain to the back side of the body, in the lumbar region close to the spine and perhaps a little lower
- if *both* right and left *iliopsoas* muscles are affected, then the pain may feel more like it is running *across* the lumbar area, rather than *vertically* (similar to a *rectus abdominis* trigger point pain referral, chapter 5), or over the upper gluteal area and sacrum (similar to a *quadratus lumborum* trigger point pain referral, chapter 6)
- other parts of the muscle (the ***iliacus***) attach to the front of the pelvis and the femur, and refer pain to the front of the thigh and groin
- pain is worse when standing, but may still be felt as a slight nagging backache when sitting or reclining
- difficulty standing up from a seated position, or an inability to straighten up enough to stand erect
- an inability to do sit-ups
- pain may be aggravated by constipation
- the most comfortable lying positions are on the side with the knees drawn up, or face-up with the knees bent
- pain unresolved by surgery may be caused by trigger points in the *iliopsoas* or the *quadratus lumborum* (chapter 6)

- in teen-age girls, if the growth of this muscle doesn't keep pace with the growth of the pelvis, it can cause appendicitis-like symptoms (pain can occur on either side, but the patient would likely only be evaluated for appendicitis if the pain was right-sided.) The *iliopsoas* may also be susceptible to easy bruising in teenage girls, even with minor injuries
- if you are taking anticoagulant drugs, this muscle may be particularly susceptible to hematomas (bruising) and can cause pain, swelling, difficulty walking, and problems with the femoral nerve (this can be diagnosed with an ultrasound)

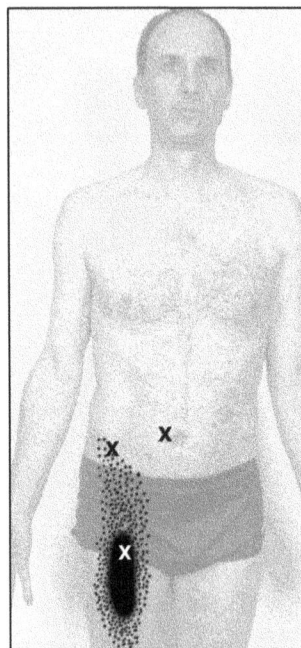

Front Referral Pattern and Trigger Points

Back Referral Pattern

Causes and Perpetuation of Trigger Points

- a fall or other sudden overload
- sitting for long periods of time with your knees at a less than 90-degree angle (knees higher than the hips), for example, in a car
- sleeping in the fetal position
- sit-ups
- tightness of the *rectus femoris* muscle (in the front of the thigh)
- pregnancy
- painful menses
- vertebrae out-of-alignment in the T10 - L1 area (for the **psoas** portion)
- L-5 vertebra out-of-alignment (for the *iliacus* portion)
- a shorter leg or small hemipelvis (either the right or left half of the pelvis)

This is a list of perpetuating factors specific only to trigger points in this muscle. For a full list of perpetuating factors that can cause and perpetuate trigger points anywhere in the body and which also apply to this muscle, please see "Appendix A" (found at the end of this book), since some may need to be addressed for lasting pain relief.

Helpful Hints

- Search for trigger points in the *quadratus lumborum* muscle (chapter 6), since the *iliopsoas* is rarely involved by itself.
- Apply moist heat over the abdomen and upper 1/3 of the thigh.
- If you are unable to stand, you may be able to crawl on your hands and knees until you are able to treat the muscles.
- When sitting, increase the angle between your thighs and trunk by leaning back against a slightly reclined backrest.
- If you must sit for periods of time, stand up frequently to stretch.
- Learn to breathe properly (see below).
- Sleep with a pillow under your knees. Avoid sleeping curled up tightly in the fetal position.
- Buy a firm mattress, and replace it every five to seven years. You can put plywood between the box springs and mattress to make it firmer.
- Don't overstretch if you do the In-Bathtub stretch (*paraspinals*, chapter 3). If you stretch by reaching toward your toes, do not overstretch by forcing it, or you can severely aggravate *iliopsoas* trigger points.
- Mis-alignments in the lumbar vertebrae and sacroiliac joint can prevent successful treatment of the *iliopsoas* muscles.
- See a specialist to be fitted for compensating lifts and pads if you have one leg shorter than the other, or a small hemipelvis (either the right or left half of the pelvis).

Self-Help Techniques

The *iliopsoas* may be providing "splinting" for other muscles (protecting other weak muscles by contracting), and if this is removed by the *iliopsoas* being relaxed, it may cause increased tightness and pain from the other muscles. All of the following muscles may need to be checked and treated first *before* treating the *iliopsoas*, or you may experience soreness and an increase in symptoms:

Check the *hamstrings* muscle group (chapter 11), since shortening of these muscles causes an unnatural tilt to the pelvis that overloads the *iliopsoas* muscles. Doctors Travell and Simons felt that treating the *hamstrings* prior to treating the *iliopsoas* was very important. Also check the *gluteus minimus* (chapter 8), *gluteus medius* (chapter 7), *gluteus maximus* (chapter 9), *paraspinal* muscles (chapter 3), and *posterior neck* muscles (self-help pressure and stretches found in chapter 3), since trigger points in the *iliopsoas* can cause and perpetuate trigger points in those other areas. All of these muscles may need to be checked for trigger points and treated first, before treating the *iliopsoas*, or you may experience soreness and an increase in symptoms.

Applying Pressure

Iliopsoas Pressure: Because these muscles are so deep, it is difficult to access them completely to apply pressure to trigger points. You will not be able to look at what you are doing at the same time as you are applying pressure, since that will cause the muscle you are trying to work on to contract, so you will have to do it by feeling with your fingers. The *iliopsoas* self-treatment will be difficult if you have long fingernails.

There are three parts of the muscle to test for tenderness and work on. Lie face-up, with something under your knees. Starting four-fingers' width away from the belly button, with your fingers back to back and the knuckles together, first press straight toward your back, then start angling in toward your spine. The position of the fingers and knuckles is very important in being able to apply sufficient pressure. Also do the same technique just above and below your belly button.

Next, hook your thumbs into the front of your pelvis, searching around the rim.

Last, check the front of your thigh, which is a little easier to reach by sitting up with your back supported to take tension off the muscle. This point is a little below the groin and about one third of the way out from the pubic area. This point is difficult to find if it is not tight and tender, but when it *is* part of the problem, a little searching will generally locate it quickly. Be sure not to press too hard in this last area, since there are major nerves and arteries located here.

Stretches

Don't overstretch if you do the In-Bathtub stretch (chapter 3). If you stretch by reaching toward your toes, don't overstretch by forcing it, or you can severely aggravate *iliopsoas* trigger points.

Abdominal Stretch: See chapter 5.

Hip-Extension Stretch: See chapter 5.

Thigh-Hip Extension Stretch: Grab onto something for support, place one leg stretched out well behind you, and bend the other leg at the knee. Gently extend your pelvis forward.

Proper Breathing Exercise: Learning to breathe properly is important for resolving trigger points in several muscles.

Place one hand on your chest and the other on your belly. When you inhale, both hands should rise. As you exhale, both hands should fall. You need to train yourself to notice when you're breathing only into your chest and make sure you start breathing into your belly.

Also See:

* Quadratus lumborum (chapter 6)
* Abdominal muscles (lower portion of the rectus abdominis, chapter 5)
* Paraspinal muscles (longissimus thoracis and multifidi, chapter 3)
* Gluteus maximus (chapter 9)
* Gluteus medius (chapter 7)

Chapter 5: Abdominals

(External Abdominal Oblique, Transversus Abdominis,
Rectus Abdominis, Pyramidalis)

Trigger points in *abdominal* muscles can cause symptoms such as projectile vomiting, loss of appetite, food intolerance, nausea, belching or burping, heartburn, pain in the bowels, diarrhea, urinary bladder spasms, testicular pain, and painful menses. These symptoms can often be confused with organ problems, but trigger points can be initiated by organ diseases and outlast the disease. You need to rule out organ diseases, and any found need to be treated for lasting relief.

Common Symptoms

- See the pictures for all the referral patterns. These pictures show common trigger points and referral patterns, but trigger points can refer pain or discomfort to the opposite side of the abdomen and even to the back.
- pain that feels like it is in an organ
- often symptoms are described as burning, fullness, bloating, swelling, or excessive gas
- forceful breathing may increase pain

Abdominal Obliques and Transversus Abdominis
- the upper trigger points may produce stomach area pain and/or heartburn and other symptoms commonly associated with a hiatal hernia, but pain is more likely to be continuous, rather than related to the timing of eating or bowel movements
- the lower points may produce urinary frequency, retention of urine, bed-wetting, chronic diarrhea, and groin and testicular pain

- frequent belching and gas, or projectile vomiting (the trigger point is likely found on the back, at or near the bottom of the rib cage)
- restricted trunk rotation

Rectus Abdominis & Pyramidalis

- in the upper portion, symptoms may include referred pain to the mid-back that crosses the back in a horizontal band, abdominal fullness, heartburn, indigestion, heart-area pain, gallbladder-area pain, peptic ulcer-like pain, gynecological-like pain, and sometimes nausea and vomiting
- around the belly button, trigger points are typically aggravated by bending over when lifting, and can cause abdominal or intestinal cramping (if your baby is colicky, try pressing points around the belly button)
- the lower 1/3 of this muscle can cause referred pain that crosses the low back and sacrum in a horizontal band, pain with menses, penis pain, diarrhea, urinary frequency, urinary retention, spasm of the urinary and detrusor sphincter muscles, and pain that *mimics* diverticulitis, kidney stones, and menstrual problems
- "McBurney's" point, usually on the right side a little way down from the level of the belly button and about three-finger's width away from the midline, can cause symptoms that mimic appendicitis. Pain often occurs when the patient is fatigued or worried, or pre-menstrually. At least 12.4% of appendixes removed are normal, and surgery does not solve the pain. In this case, pain is likely due instead to trigger points. However, since a ruptured appendix is life-threatening, you may not have time to rule out trigger points. *With any sudden onset of abdominal pain, go to the emergency room immediately for evaluation*, including a blood test for infection. If you end up having surgery and it did not solve all or part of the problem, search for trigger points.
- "*Rectus Abdominis* syndrome" is entrapment of an anterior branch of a spinal nerve, causing lower abdominal and pelvic pain that simulates gynecological problems in women
- The pyramidalis causes referred pain close to the midline, between the belly button and the top of the pubic bone

Sample Trigger Points

Sample Referral Patterns

> **Sample rectus abdominis referral patterns, but all of these can occur at any level of the back.**

McBurney's point

Painful menses

Pyramidalis

Causes and Perpetuation of Trigger Points

- poor posture such as bending over for long periods of time, your back not being supported, or rotating to one side to see your computer screen
- improper conditioning (i.e., too many sit-ups too soon)
- trying to hold your abdomen in continuously
- a tight belt
- emotional stress
- overall fatigue
- straining due to constipation
- exposure to cold temperatures (due to tensing up)
- direct trauma to the abdominal area, including surgeries such as appendectomies or hysterectomies
- viral infections
- trigger points can be initiated by organ diseases such as a peptic ulcer, intestinal parasites (such as *Entamoeba histolytica*, and beef or fish tapeworms), dysentery (diarrhea caused most likely by drinking unclean water), diverticulosis, diverticulitis, and gallstones, and trigger points may cause symptoms that outlast the organ disease even after resolution of the disease
- a short leg or small hemipelvis (either the right or left half of the pelvis)

This is a list of perpetuating factors specific only to trigger points in <u>these</u> muscles. For a full list of perpetuating factors that can cause and perpetuate trigger points anywhere in the body and which also apply to these muscles, please see "Appendix A" (found at the end of this book), since some may need to be addressed for lasting pain relief.

Helpful Hints

- Make sure your belt, waistband, or pantyhose elastic isn't compressing the muscles. If something is leaving a mark on your skin, it is too tight.
- Use a lumbar support everywhere you sit. Modify or replace your mis-fitting furniture. Your knees should fit under your desk, and the chair needs to be close enough that you can lean against your backrest. Your elbows should rest on either your work surface or armrests at the same height. Your elbows and forearms should rest evenly on the armrests. Your computer screen should be directly in front of you, and the copy attached to the side of the screen, so that you may look directly forward as much as possible. Take frequent breaks.
- Don't try to hold your abdomen in to make it flat. This actually has the opposite effect, since the chronic tension will form trigger points which cause the muscle fibers to stop their proper contraction function, and allow the abdomen to go slack due to an inability to condition the muscles.
- Learn proper breathing techniques (chapter 4).
- Laughter is a good exercise for *abdominal* muscles.
- Treat the causes of stress and emotional upsets.
- Too many sit-ups can not only cause trigger points in the *abdominal* muscles, but can lead to satellite trigger points in the *diaphragm* muscle as well (the muscle that divides the thoracic cavity and the abdominal cavity)
- Learn proper conditioning techniques, either with the help of a physical therapist or other trained specialist who knows how to modify an activity for your set of circumstances. Don't overdo conditioning exercises. You shouldn't do activities that are painful, or make you sore later. It is better to add repetitions and increase weights *slowly* so that you make steady progress, rather than hurt yourself and have to stop until you are well again.
- Treat the cause of constipation. Acupuncture and herbs are very successful at treating constipation.
- Head-forward posture can be a result of trigger points in the *upper rectus abdominis* muscle.
- Treat organ diseases such as ulcers, gallstones, parasites, and diverticulitis.
- Scars left from surgeries usually cause numerous trigger points in the surrounding muscles, so check for trigger points around any abdominal scars. Acupuncture scar treatments are very effective for treating these trigger points, even years after the surgery.

Self-Help Techniques

Abdominal pain may be trigger point referral from the *paraspinal* muscles (chapter 3), and pain in the back may be referred from trigger points in the *abdominal* muscles, so you should check both sets of muscles. Gastrointestinal pain and cramping, and nausea and belching may also be due to trigger points in the *paraspinal* muscles (chapter 3). Lower abdominal pain, tenderness, and muscle spasming may also come from trigger points located in the vaginal wall (see *pelvic floor* muscles, chapter 12).

Applying Pressure

Abdominal Pressure: Lying face-up, use your fingers to apply pressure to sensitive points in the entire abdominal area. You may find it easier if you have a pillow under your knees. Be sure to check all the way from the bottom rib to the top of the pubic bone, and out to the sides. When working on the top edge of the pubic bone, press down toward your feet rather than toward your back. You may combine this with applying hot packs or sitting in a warm bath.

Stretches

Abdominal Stretch: Use something round such as a large inflatable therapeutic exercise ball (from a chiropractor or physical therapist) or a concrete form tube (from a building supply store). Lie face-up over it with your arms outstretched over your head and touch your palms to the floor. Be careful not to fall over, and don't do this stretch if you are elderly or pregnant. I find the concrete form tube easier to use, since you can't roll off to the side. You may not be able to perform this stretch if you have back problems.

Hip-Extension Stretch: As an alternative to the Abdominal Stretch, lie face-down on a flat surface, such as the floor. Using your arms, push your torso off of the surface with your head looking straight ahead at the wall, but keep your pelvis on the surface. If you can only rest on your elbows, you will still get a stretch. Breathe deeply to expand your abdomen. You may not be able to do this stretch if you have neck or shoulder girdle problems**.**

Exercises

Pelvic Tilt Exercise: The pelvic tilt strengthens the *rectus abdominis*. Once trigger points have been inactivated for a few weeks, you may add this conditioning exercise. With this exercise, be sure to rest between each repetition for an equal amount of time it took to perform the repetition.

Lie face-up with your knees bent, with one hand over your lower abdomen and one hand above your navel.

First flatten out the lumbar area of your back against the floor, which brings the two hands closer together.

Then push your butt off the floor so only your feet and mid to upper back are still on the floor—the hands should come even closer together. If your hands get further apart, you are arching your back rather than flattening it correctly.

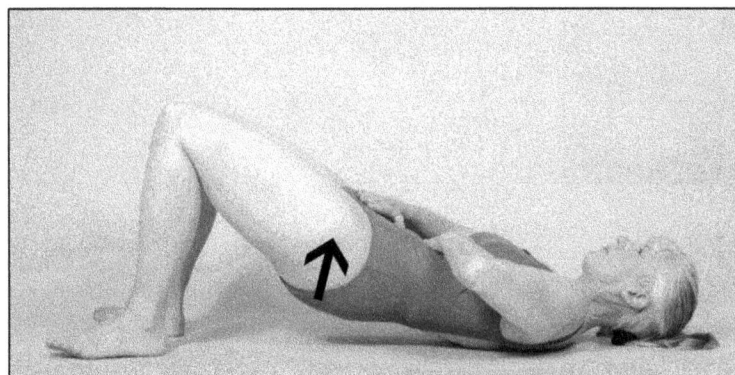

Finally, roll back down to relax on the floor and take a deep breath.

Also See:

*   Paraspinal muscles (chapter 3)

You may also need to search for trigger points in the *serratus anterior*, *diaphragm*, and *adductor muscles of the hip*, since trigger points in those muscles can either cause similar pain referral patterns or may affect or be affected by *abdominal* trigger points in some way.

Since trigger points in these muscles don't directly cause lower back and gluteal pain, they are not addressed in this book. If you can't relieve your pain with the self-help techniques in this book after six to eight weeks, you may wish to consider whether you need to treat trigger points in these additional muscles, or if you still have perpetuating factors to resolve. Go to the end of this book for other books by the author that provide self-treatment techniques of muscles not covered in this book.

Differential Diagnosis: *If you are experiencing sudden abdominal pain, go to the emergency room!* Abdominal pain more likely due to trigger points in the rectus abdominis muscle will exhibit palpable nodules and ropiness in the band of muscle down the middle of the abdomen. Abdominal pain more likely due to appendicitis will exhibit a more generalized, board-like rigidity in the entire abdominal musculature. Your health care provider will conduct other tests to evaluate you for appendicitis, including a blood test. I had one patient who suffered from low-grade abdominal pain that was helped minimally by massage and acupuncture. After several months, she had her appendix removed on the advice of a health care provider. Her pain was relieved, and it was determined she had a subclinical chronic irritation of her appendix with fibrous tissues, even though it was not diseased.

Once a health care provider has ruled out appendicitis, you may also need to be evaluated for a peptic ulcer, colitis, painful rib syndrome, urinary tract disease, fibromyalgia, a hiatal hernia, gastric carcinoma, kidney or gallstones, an inguinal hernia, hepatitis, pancreatitis, gynecological disorders, diverticulosis, an umbilical hernia, thoracic or upper lumbar nerve root irritation, costochondritis, ascariasis, epilepsy, and rectus abdominis hematoma. Pain in the upper abdomen may be caused by Tietze's syndrome or slipping rib syndrome. You may need to see a chiropractor or osteopathic physician to be evaluated for pubic and innominate dysfunctions or for vertebral and rib misalignments.

Chapter 6: Quadratus Lumborum
(and Iliolumbar Ligament)

In the United States, low back pain causes some degree of work disability in 10-15% of adults per year, costing billions of dollars in sick days, reduced productivity, and health insurance claims. People with disabling low back pain receive more than $3 billion per year just in disability payments. Recognition and treatment of trigger points could reduce these sums substantially. Trigger points in the *quadratus lumborum* muscle are responsible for roughly 30% of sacral-gluteal pain.

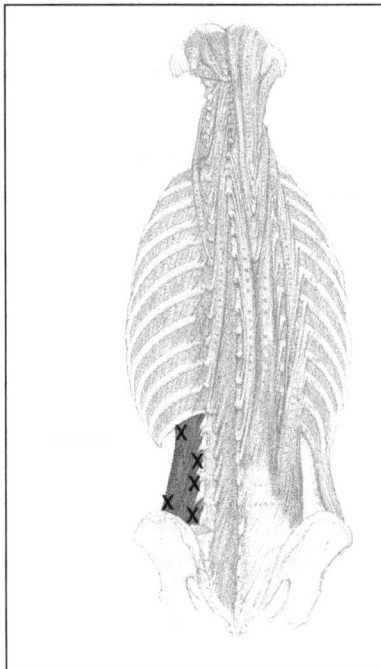

Back view of trunk

Common Symptoms

- depending on the location of the trigger points, pain can be referred to various places in the gluteal area, the sacrum, over the hip joint and surrounding area, and even around the front to the groin area, testis, scrotum, and the lower abdomen (see the pictures for the referral patterns)
- pain is usually deep and aching, but can be sharp or stabbing with movement
- possibly unbearable pain with standing or sitting upright, but you may be able to crawl on your hands and knees
- pain with climbing stairs
- rotating your trunk, or leaning to the opposite side is very painful
- rolling onto your side, getting up, or getting out of a chair may be extremely painful or impossible
- pain can be so intolerable you cannot lie on the affected side
- you may be unable to bear weight on the affected side

- coughing or sneezing can cause unbearable pain temporarily
- range-of-motion can be restricted with bending forward
- pain over the sacroiliac joint (where the sacrum and big pelvic bone join) and greater trochanter (hip joint) can be mistaken for joint dysfunction
- constant pain eventually causes fatigue and probably depression
- a small number of patients may experience a "lightning bolt" of pain down the front of the thigh in a narrow band
- possibly "heaviness of the hips," calf cramping, and burning sensations in the legs and feet
- a "sciatica" type of pain distribution that may be reproduced by pressing on *quadratus lumborum* trigger points and possibly some *gluteus minimus* trigger points ("pseudo-sciatica")

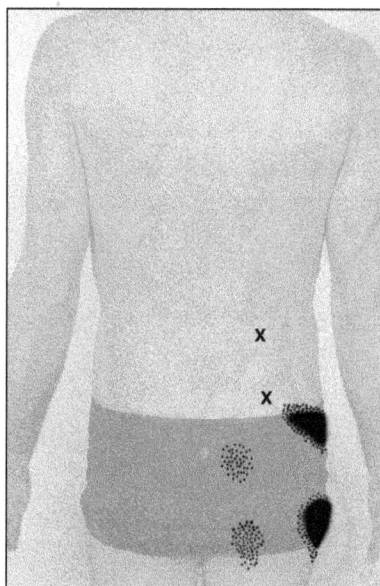

Deep fibers	**Superficial fibers**	**Superficial fibers front referral pattern**

- the *iliolumbar ligament* can refer pain locally around the 4th and 5th lumbar vertebrae, but can also cause pain that feels like it is deep in the hip joint, in the groin area, and diffusely over the front of the thigh

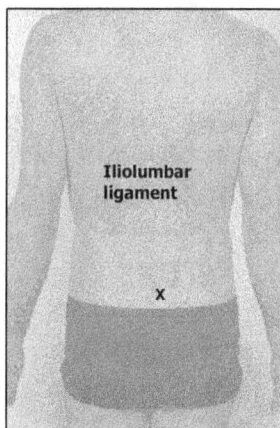

Iliolumbar ligament

Causes and Perpetuation of Trigger Points

- trauma, such as an auto accident
- awkward movements, such as lifting something heavy, especially when your trunk is rotated at the same time, or trying to rise out of a low chair, car, or bed
- attempting to put on pants, socks, and shoes while standing
- a near fall, where you catch yourself
- a repetitive strain from gardening, washing floors, lifting heavy objects, or walking or running on slanted surfaces such as a beach or road
- leaning forward over a desk, sink, or other work surface
- weak *abdominal* muscles (chapter 5)
- mattresses that are too old or too soft, or sleeping next to someone who is heavier and trying to avoid rolling into them
- walking in a cast
- one leg *anatomically* shorter than the other with as little as 1/8" difference (if this were the case you would probably stand with one foot forward, with your weight on the short foot, or with your pelvis shifted to the shorter side, and you probably would have pain with walking and standing). This does *not* refer to the "short leg" terminology chiropractors often use to describe the effect of vertebrae being out-of-alignment.
- a small hemipelvis (either the right or left half of the pelvis), and sitting aggravates the pain
- short upper arms, causing you to lean to one side to use armrests, and sitting aggravates the pain

This is a list of perpetuating factors specific only to trigger points in <u>this</u> muscle. For a full list of perpetuating factors that can cause and perpetuate trigger points anywhere in the body and which also apply to this muscle, please see "Appendix A" (found at the end of this book), since some may need to be addressed for lasting pain relief.

Helpful Hints

- Some of my patients have assumed their pain in the lumbar region meant they had a kidney infection. Symptoms of a kidney infection include a high fever and chills. ***If you are experiencing those symptoms, go to the emergency room immediately***. Otherwise, check for trigger points and see if you can get relief.
- Don't assume that a finding of bone spurs or narrowing of the lumbar disc space is causing the pain, since many people who have these do not have pain, and vice versa. Always assume trigger points are at least a part of the problem.
- You may find relief by lying on your back or side. Using a pillow to modify the tilt of your hips or placing it under your knees may be helpful. If you are comfortable lying on your side, place a pillow in front of your legs and put your upper leg on top of it.
- Always be sure to have proper lumbar support in all sitting locations, including your car.
- Sit while putting on pants, socks, and shoes.
- Avoid any heavy lifting, and if you must lift something, be sure to bend at the knees, keep your torso straight, and keep the object close to your body.

- Stand up straight, rather than bending over sinks and work surfaces. If you must lean over something, keep it brief and support yourself with a free hand.
- When standing up from a chair, slide your butt to the front of the chair, turn your entire body a little sideways, put one foot under the front edge of the chair, then stand with the torso erect so that your thighs take the load. You can use your hands to assist you if necessary. Sit down in the opposite sequence.
- When climbing stairs or a ladder, rotate your entire body 45-degrees and keep your back straight.
- Gardeners should sit on a stool about eight to ten inches high, and take frequent breaks.
- Buy a firm mattress, and replace it every five to seven years. You can put plywood between the box springs and mattress to make it firmer.
- Don't carry a wallet in your back pocket, as this tilts your pelvis when you sit on it.
- Make sure your muscles don't get chilled, especially at night.
- If you must wear a walking cast due to a broken bone, get a shoe for the opposite foot with a sole that matches the height of the bottom of the cast.
- See a specialist for corrective orthotics, and compensating lifts and pads if necessary. If an anatomical leg length inequality is not corrected, it can contribute to osteoarthritis of the hip and lumbar spine. Symptoms from an anatomical leg length inequality may not show up until it is brought on by an acute trauma, such as a car accident. If you use compensating lifts, you must use them all the time, in all shoes, and not go barefoot. (Evaluation of various body asymmetries is discussed in detail in: Janet G. Travell, M.D., and David G. Simons, M.D., *Myofascial Pain and Dysfunction: The Trigger Point Manual, The Lower Extremities vol. 2* (Baltimore: Williams & Wilkins, 1992), pp. 41-63.
- If you are getting an anatomical leg-length inequity corrected with lifts, start with a thin lift and gradually use thicker ones until the proper lift height is reached.
- Armrests can be corrected by taping sponges or towels to the armrests.

Self-Help Techniques

Always do the self-treatment on *both* sides! It is rare that only one side is involved, especially in the lumbar and gluteal muscles. Check the *gluteus medius* muscle (chapter 7), since trigger points in that muscle can activate *quadratus lumborum* trigger points. Trigger points in the *gluteus medius* (chapter 7) and *gluteus minimus* (chapter 8) can cause weakness in the *quadratus lumborum*. Consider acupuncture for treatment of the *quadratus lumborum*, since needles are better able to penetrate down to the muscle than massage.

Wrapping your hands around the sides of your waist and pressing downward on the top of your pelvis may give enough temporary relief to allow some movement, as may using your thumbs to apply pressure to the muscle itself.

Applying Pressure

Paraspinal Pressure: As part of the quadratus lumborum self-treatment, work on the *paraspinal* muscles (chapter 3), because most of the time those muscles are also involved to some extent.

Quadratus Lumborum Pressure: When you get to the lumbar area, most people have enough of a curve that they might need to move to the floor and use a tennis ball or baseball, but make sure this is not too hard for you (see the general guidelines in chapter 1). Don't use a softball since it is too large. You may use your hand to move the ball, searching for trigger points in the lumbar area. *Do not press your back onto the ball and if you have been diagnosed with bulging or herniated discs, be very careful not to get too close to the spine!*

Iliolumbar Ligament Pressure: The *iliolumbar ligament* is in a small dip between the fifth lumbar vertebra and the rim of your pelvis. It is helpful to locate it with your thumb first. Lying face-up with your knees bent, on a hard surface such as a wood or linoleum floor or on a very thin carpet, use a golf ball and your body weight to give you pressure. If this is not enough pressure, put the calf of the same side on top of the opposite knee. You may also wish to continue down a little further onto the top part of the sacrum, in order to get the S_1 multifidi (see chapter 3 for a picture of the *multifidi* muscles).

Demonstrating location of iliolumbar ligament

Stretches

Supine Self-Stretch: Lie face-up with your knees bent and with your hands behind your head; if you don't put your hands behind your head, you will not get the stretch. Place one leg over the other knee, and use that leg to gently pull the knee down toward the floor. You should feel the stretch in the lumbar and gluteal areas. Then slip the leg off of the knee, return to neutral position, and repeat on the opposite side. You may repeat this a few times on each side. Follow with the Hip-Hike Stretch below.

Hip-Hike Stretch: Lie face-up with your legs out straight. Place your hands on your hips, and as you breathe in, stretch one leg down so your pelvis tilts down on that side and you are feeling a stretch in the lumbar area. Exhale as you return to the neutral position. Repeat on the other side.

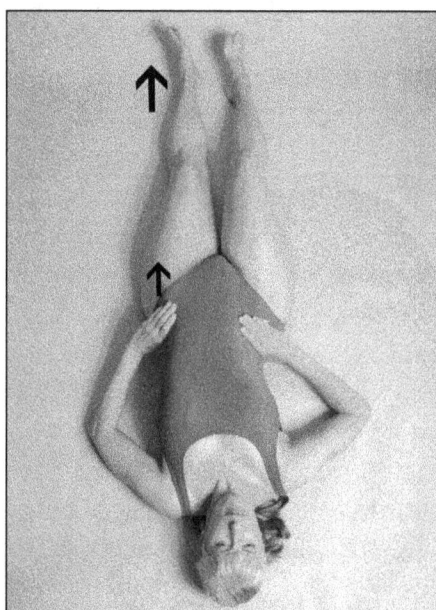

Exercises

Supine Self-Stretch with Resistance: Once trigger points have been inactivated for a few weeks and are no longer causing referred pain, during the Supine Self-Stretch you may briefly apply resistance to provide an additional stretch. While you are using the left leg to stretch the right side, briefly use the right knee to push up against the left leg, then relax, taking up the slack in the stretch, and repeat. Do the same on the opposite side.

Also See:

* Paraspinals (chapter 3)
* Iliopsoas (chapter 4)
* Abdominals (chapter 5)
* Gluteus medius (primary or satellite trigger points, chapter 7)
* Gluteus minimus (satellite trigger points, chapter 8)

You may also need to search for trigger points in the *latissimus dorsi*, since trigger points in this muscle can either cause similar pain referral patterns or may affect or be affected by *quadratus lumborum* trigger points in some way.

Since trigger points in this muscle don't directly cause lower back and gluteal pain, it is not addressed in this book. If you can't relieve your pain with the self-help techniques in this book after six to eight weeks, you may wish to consider whether you need to treat trigger points in this additional muscle, or if you still have perpetuating factors to resolve. Go to the end of this book for other books by the author that provide self-treatment techniques of muscles not covered in this book.

Differential Diagnosis: If you are unable to relieve your symptoms with trigger point self-help techniques, you may need to see a health care provider to rule out spinal tumors, myasthenia gravis, gallstones, liver disease, kidney stones, urinary tract problems, intra-abdominal infections, intestinal parasites, diverticulitis, an aortic aneurysm, and multiple sclerosis. See a chiropractor or osteopathic physician for evaluation of vertebrae out of alignment and sacroiliac joint subluxation.

Be sure to address any perpetuating factors when low back pain has persisted for more than a few weeks or doesn't respond more than temporarily to trigger point treatment. Particularly examine vitamin and other nutritional deficiencies, organ dysfunction and disease especially thyroid inadequacies, acute or chronic viral, bacterial, or parasitic infections, emotional factors, or active allergies with a high histamine level. Go to the end of this book, "Appendix A," for detailed information on perpetuating factors.

Chapter 7: Gluteus Medius

Pain from trigger points in the *gluteus medius* muscle is frequently referred to as low back pain, or lumbago. This muscle is essential for endurance and full strength in walking and other more vigorous activities.

Common Symptoms

- referred pain over the sacrum, along the sacroiliac joint, and over the rest of the buttocks, depending on the site of the trigger point
- pain with walking, especially if you have a short big toe and longer second toe
- difficulty sleeping on the affected side, and possibly on your back
- pain with sitting in a slumped position
- trigger points may contribute to neck pain and headaches
- TrP 3 is very common in office workers and runners

Trigger Point #1   *Trigger Point #2*   *Trigger Point #3*

Causes and Perpetuation of Trigger Points
- sudden falls
- sports injuries
- running, long tennis matches, or aerobic exercises
- long walks on a sandy beach
- riding an upright bicycle, such as an exercise bike
- standing with your weight shifted to one leg for long periods of time
- sleeping in the fetal position
- sitting in a chair that is too low
- holding your head too far forward

- sitting on a wallet in your back pocket
- injections of medications into the muscle, especially irritant medications
- one leg *anatomically* shorter than the other (this does *not* refer to the "short leg" terminology chiropractors often use to describe the effect of vertebrae being out-of-alignment)
- a short big toe and longer second toe (causes excessive pronation - standing with your weight more toward the outside of your feet)
- sacroiliac joint out-of-alignment (the joint where the sacrum and big pelvic bone join)

This is a list of perpetuating factors specific only to trigger points in this muscle. For a full list of perpetuating factors that can cause and perpetuate trigger points anywhere in the body and which also apply to this muscle, please see "Appendix A" (found at the end of this book), since some may need to be addressed for lasting pain relief.

Helpful Hints

- When sleeping on your side, place a pillow between your knees. The most comfortable position may be lying on the unaffected side, tilted back with your torso supported by a pillow behind you.
- Sit down while putting clothing and shoes on your lower body.
- Avoid sitting for too long in one position, and don't cross your legs. Setting a timer across the room ensures that you get up periodically to turn it off.
- Don't carry a wallet in your back pocket.
- If you have a short big toe and long second toe, get corrective orthotics to prevent pronation.
- If you get injections in this muscle, have the health care provider select sites that are not tender.

Self-Help Techniques

If you only get temporary relief with self-work, check the *quadratus lumborum* (chapter 6), since trigger points in that muscle can cause and keep trigger points in the *gluteus medius* activated. Also, see a chiropractor or osteopathic physician to check the sacroiliac joint and lumbar vertebrae for alignment problems. Also search for trigger points in the *piriformis* muscle (chapter 10), since it frequently contains trigger points concurrently with the *gluteus medius* muscle. If you continue to have pain after a back surgery intended to correct pain, search the entire gluteal area for potential trigger points.

Applying Pressure

Paraspinal Pressure: Tightness in the opposite *paraspinal* muscles (chapter 3) can tilt and rotate the pelvis, causing pain in the hip joint and trigger points in the *gluteal* muscles. Be sure to work on the *paraspinals* first (*both* sides), and then the *gluteal* muscles on both right *and* left sides.

Gluteus Medius Pressure: Common trigger points in the *gluteus medius* are higher up than most people think, so they are easy to miss. It's also usually tender lower down too, so you may think you have found the muscle, when in fact you have missed it. If you wear briefs or pants that come to your waist, the trigger points are just below your underpants line or your belt, just below the rim of the pelvis. They are also out to the side, so you have to work under the whole rim.

Demonstrating location of gluteus medius trigger points

Lie face-up and place a ball close to your sacrum (the bony triangle in between the last lumbar vertebrae and the tailbone). Start working your way outward by moving the ball with your hand, following the rim of the pelvis. Keep going until you get all the way out to the side, to ensure that you have searched the entire muscle.

Stretches

Abductor Stretch: Lie on your bed with the front of your body next to the edge. With the leg on the bed slightly bent, drop the top leg over the edge in front of you, using gravity to give you a stretch.

Then, lying with your back to the edge of the bed, drop the top leg over the edge behind you. With both stretches, use deep breathing to assist in lengthening the stretch.

Also See:
* Piriformis (chapter 10)
* Gluteus minimus (chapter 8)
* Gluteus maximus (chapter 9)
* Quadratus lumborum (chapter 6)

You may also need to search for trigger points in the *tensor fasciae latae*, since trigger points in this muscle can either cause similar pain referral patterns or may affect or be affected by *gluteus medius* trigger points in some way.

Since trigger points in this muscle don't directly cause lower back and gluteal pain, it is not addressed in this book. If you can't relieve your pain with the self-help techniques in this book after six to eight weeks, you may wish to consider whether you need to treat trigger points in this additional muscle, or if you still have perpetuating factors to resolve. Go to the end of this book for other books by the author that provide self-treatment techniques of muscles not covered in this book.

> **Differential Diagnosis:** If you are unable to relieve your symptoms with trigger point self-help techniques, you may need to see a health care provider to rule out intermittent claudication (narrowing of some of the major arteries) if you or your family has a history of heart or circulatory system problems, since that condition could cause trigger points in the gluteus medius and tensor fasciae latae muscles.

Chapter 8: Gluteus Minimus

Referred pain from trigger points in the *gluteus minimus* frequently gets diagnosed by both patients and practitioners as "sciatic pain," because of the distribution pattern down the side and back of the legs. At least 80% of pain down the leg comes from trigger point referral, not from "pinched nerves," a herniated disc, or stenosis in a lumbar vertebra (narrowing of either the big hole in the vertebra that the spinal cord goes through, or narrowing of the smaller holes the nerves travel out through). Since "sciatica" is usually assumed to be caused by compression of a nerve, pain referrals from trigger points are probably more aptly called "pseudo-sciatica."

I have found that if the pain is truly coming from a disc or problem with a lumbar vertebra, the patient usually draws a referral pattern that starts as a thin line coming from a very specific spot on one side of a lumbar vertebra, and then continues into the gluteal area and down the leg. The pain is usually sharper and intense. If the pain referral starts in the gluteal area and not a pinpoint spot in the lumbar area, it is likely caused by trigger points in either the *gluteus minimus* or *piriformis* muscles (chapter 10). If it does start next to a vertebra, you need to see a health care provider and get an MRI to be evaluated for disc problems and stenosis.

Back view of gluteal area and thigh

Common Symptoms

- the anterior portion of the muscle (on your side, under the seam of your pants) refers pain down the side of the leg to the ankle, and possibly to a spot on the backside of your buttocks
- the posterior portion of the muscle is part way between the side and the backside, and refers pain over the gluteal area and down the back of the leg into the calf
- hip pain may cause a limp with walking
- pain with sleeping on the affected side, severe enough to wake you
- difficulty rising out of a chair after sitting for a while
- difficulty in finding a comfortable position standing, walking, or lying down
- pain with running or hiking

Gluteus Minimus Anterior   *Gluteus Minimus Posterior*

Causes and Perpetuation of Trigger Points

- sudden or chronic overuse
- sitting with a wallet in your back pocket
- standing for long periods with your weight shifted to one side or with your feet too close together
- sitting for too long, especially when driving
- a fall

- walking or running too far or too fast, especially on rough ground
- overuse while playing tennis, racquetball, or handball
- chilling of the muscle or the body as a whole
- walking with a limp from an injury
- injections of medications, especially irritants, can cause pain that lasts for months
- the sacroiliac joint out-of-alignment (the joint where the sacrum and big pelvic bone join)
- a nerve root irritation
- a small hemipelvis (either the right or left half of the pelvis)
- obesity tends to overload these muscles

This is a list of perpetuating factors specific only to trigger points in <u>this</u> muscle. For a full list of perpetuating factors that can cause and perpetuate trigger points anywhere in the body and which also apply to this muscle, please see "Appendix A" (found at the end of this book), since some may need to be addressed for lasting pain relief.

Helpful Hints

- Runners and avid hikers usually have *gluteus minimus* trigger points. If you have located trigger points with the self-help techniques, back off on your runs or hikes until the trigger points have improved dramatically. You can then *slowly* increase your mileage, staying out of the pain zone. I recommend doing the ball self-work and ample stretching before and after the run.
- Don't carry a wallet in your back pocket.
- If you must stand for long periods, stand with your feet apart and shift your weight frequently from one foot to the other.
- If you sit for long periods, move around the room every 15-20 minutes. A timer set across the room ensures that you will get up periodically to turn it off.
- Keep your body, and particularly these muscles, warm.
- Sleep with a pillow between your legs.
- If you are obese, don't over-do exercising these muscles until trigger points have been inactivated and strength is built-up gradually. Walk with a wider stance.
- See a chiropractor or osteopathic physician to check the sacroiliac joint and lumbar vertebrae for alignment problems.
- If you have a small hemipelvis (either the right or left half of the pelvis) or other structural imbalance, see a specialist for compensating lifts and pads.
- Acupuncture will help with disc problems, but will only help with the pain from stenosis. It will not affect the stenosis, which may require surgery. These surgeries have gotten very sophisticated in recent years, and usually have you back on your feet the day after the surgery.
- If you receive muscular injections, avoid this muscle. Inject into the *gluteus medius* (chapter 7) and *deltoid* muscles, since they are less prone to developing trigger points.
- If pain remains after a laminectomy surgery, check the *gluteus minimus* for trigger points.

Self-Help Techniques

If you only get temporary relief with the self-help techniques, check the *quadratus lumborum* (chapter 6), since trigger points in that muscle can cause and keep trigger points in the *gluteus minimus* activated.

Applying Pressure

Paraspinal Pressure: Tightness in the opposite *paraspinal* muscles (chapter 3) can tilt and rotate the pelvis, causing pain in the hip joint and trigger points in the *gluteal* muscles. Be sure to work on the *paraspinals* first (*both* sides), and then the *gluteal* muscles on both right *and* left sides.

Gluteus Minimus Pressure: Be sure to work on the *gluteus minimus* muscles on both right *and* left sides of your body. Common trigger points in the *gluteus minimus* are found in the upper third of the back of your gluteal area, to over on the side between your hip joint and the top of your pelvis.

Gluteus Minimus Anterior
Demonstrating location to use ball

Gluteus Minimus Posterior
Demonstrating location to use ball

Lying face-up on a tennis ball, move the ball with your hand while searching for trigger points.

Start moving gradually out onto your side. By the time you work on the entire *gluteus minimus* muscle, you will be lying on your side. Many patients make the mistake of not getting far enough forward. If you are working over the seam of your pants, you are reaching all the points; otherwise, keep searching further forward.

Stretches

Gluteus Minimus Stretch, Anterior Muscle Portion: To stretch the *anterior* fibers of the *gluteus minimus* muscle, lie on your side on the edge of the bed with your back flush to the edge. Allow your top leg to drop behind you, off the edge. Allow gravity to give you a stretch. If you want more of a stretch, put the heel of your opposite leg on the side of your calf. Then move your heel closer to your knee for an even greater stretch.

Gluteus Minimus Stretch, Posterior Muscle Portion: To stretch the *posterior* fibers of the *gluteus minimus* muscle, lie on your side and position yourself at the foot of the bed with the top leg out over the end and slightly forward of the line of your trunk, with your toes slightly rotated toward the floor. Your bottom leg is bent at more than 90°, so that it is still mostly on the bed. Let gravity give you a stretch.

Also See:
*   Piriformis (chapter 10)
*   Gluteus medius (chapter 7)
*   Quadratus lumborum (chapter 6)
*   Gluteus maximus (chapter 9)

If the pain feels deep in the hip joint, it is more likely coming from trigger points in the *tensor fasciae latae* muscle instead of the *gluteus minimus*. If pain is over the sacrum (the bony triangle between the spine and the tailbone) or the sacroiliac joint, trigger points are more likely located in the *gluteus medius* (chapter 7).

You may also need to search for trigger points in the *tensor fasciae latae, vastus lateralis,* and *peroneus longus*, since trigger points in those muscles can either cause similar pain referral patterns or may affect or be affected by *gluteus minimus* trigger points in some way.

Since trigger points in these muscles don't directly cause lower back and gluteal pain, they are not addressed in this book. If you can't relieve your pain with the self-help techniques in this book after six to eight weeks, you may wish to consider whether you need to treat trigger points in these additional muscles, or if you still have perpetuating factors to resolve. Go to the end of this book for other books by the author that provide self-treatment techniques of muscles not covered in this book.

Differential Diagnosis: If the pain is very localized over the hip joint or perhaps from the buttocks down the side to the knee, it may be *trochanteric bursitis*, which is inflammation of a fluid-filled sack over the bone that allows the gluteus minimus tendon to glide over the bony prominence. The hip joint will be very tender to pressure, and applying pressure reproduces the symptoms. Gluteus minimus trigger points can also be misdiagnosed as bursitis, so it is always worth checking the surrounding muscles for trigger points and subsequent relief. Since, in every case of *true* bursitis that I have treated, the gluteus minimus muscle was also tight, I suspect tightness and trigger points are a causative factor for the bursitis. Acupuncture can treat bursitis: I lay the patient on their side and place four to five needles around the bursa and one in the center, which is called *surround the dragon*. I also needle points along the gallbladder meridian, in addition to any trigger points that are contributing to the irritation of the bursa.

Chapter 9: Gluteus Maximus

The *gluteus maximus* is a powerful muscle used for running, jumping, climbing stairs, hiking uphill, swimming, and rising from a seated position. Its large size and fiber orientation is what allows us to stand upright on two legs, and is one of the features that distinguishes humans from other animals including other primates. It can be more than one inch in thickness.

Common Symptoms

- referred pain in the gluteal region, the lower part of the sacrum, sacroiliac joint, and/or tailbone, mostly very close to where the trigger points are located
- the most common trigger points are found next to the sacrum (the bony triangle below the spine), next to the tailbone, and a little further out along the bottom curve of the butt
- the trigger point along the bottom curve of the butt is the most common one, and can refer pain deep within the buttock, or it may feel like a nail pressing on the bone when you are sitting in a hard seat
- pain may feel like it is in the tailbone when sitting, though the tailbone does not touch the chair and the trigger point is really off to the side a little
- pain is aggravated by walking uphill, especially if you are bent forward
- pain with swimming, especially in cold water
- restricted range-of-motion when combined with *hamstring* tightness (chapter 11)

Causes and Perpetuation of Trigger Points
- a fall or near-fall, as your muscles contract to prevent the fall
- a direct blow to the muscle
- walking uphill for a long time period while leaning forward
- standing with your head too far forward

- sitting for too long in one position, particularly if you are reclining and your legs are straight
- sitting on a wallet in your back pocket
- sleeping on one side with the upper leg pulled up toward the chest and no pillow support underneath it
- sleeping on your back with your legs straight for long periods of time
- swimming, especially the crawl stroke and possibly the breast stroke
- leg lifts in either the standing or lying positions
- frequently bending over and lifting
- the sacroiliac joint being out-of-alignment (where the sacrum and the big pelvic bone join)
- a shorter big toe and longer second toe
- intramuscular injections, especially with an irritant medication

This is a list of perpetuating factors specific only to trigger points in <u>this</u> muscle. For a full list of perpetuating factors that can cause and perpetuate trigger points anywhere in the body and which also apply to this muscle, please see "Appendix A" (found at the end of this book), since some may need to be addressed for lasting pain relief.

Helpful Hints

- Don't sit for more than 15-20 minutes at a time. Walk around briefly before sitting again. Setting a timer across the room will help you to remember to take breaks.
- Place a pillow under your knees if you sleep on your back. When lying on your side, place a pillow between your legs.
- Leaning forward over work surfaces or sinks and hiking uphill should be limited until trigger points are inactivated.
- Don't put a wallet in your back pocket.
- Lifting properly requires bending at the knees, but this places a greater load on the *gluteus maximus*, so avoid lifting until trigger points are inactivated. If you must lift, bend down on one knee, then place your hand on your thigh to assist you in rising again. When getting up from a chair, place your hand on your thigh to assist you.
- If you swim, replace the crawl and breast strokes with the backstroke or sidestroke.
- See a physical therapist or other specialist for postural re-training if necessary.
- A true *anatomical* leg-length inequality of 1/4 inch or more needs to be corrected with a compensating lift (this does *not* refer to the "short leg" terminology chiropractors often use to describe the effect of vertebrae being out-of-alignment).
- If you have a short big toe and long second toe, get corrective orthotics to prevent pronation (standing with your weight more on the outside of your feet).
- See a chiropractor or osteopathic physician to see if your sacroiliac joint needs to be adjusted.

Self-Help Techniques

Applying Pressure

Paraspinal Pressure: Tightness in the opposite *paraspinal* muscles (chapter 3) can tilt and rotate the pelvis, causing pain in the hip joint and trigger points in the gluteal muscles. Be sure to work on the *paraspinals* first (*both* sides), and then the gluteal muscles on both right *and* left sides.

Gluteus Maximus Pressure: Lying face-up, use a tennis ball on the bed to search for trigger points in the gluteal area. In particular, search along the edge of the sacrum (the bony triangle below the spine). Be sure to work toward the bottom of the butt.

Demonstrating location to use ball

You may find the lower trigger points are easier to access by leaning against a padded surface such as a couch arm, where you can get pressure on the lower curve of the buttocks and near the tailbone.

Stretches

Low Back Stretching Exercise: See chapter 3 for this stretch, which also benefits the *gluteus maximus* muscle. Eventually, over time, you should be able to bring your thigh all the way to your chest without pain.

Abdominal Stretch: If the *rectus abdominis* (chapter 5) and *iliopsoas* (chapter 4) muscles contain trigger points, releasing the *gluteus maximus* can cause them to cramp. If this happens, you will need to stretch those muscles.

Exercises

The *gluteus maximus* muscle is not used while riding a stationary bike. It is used only minimally with an increased workload and pedaling rate while bicycling outdoors, or with normal walking. This means that to condition the *gluteus maximus* once trigger points are inactivated, you must swim, hike uphill, jump, or do some other vigorous activity. Conditioning the *gluteus maximus* requires that you keep your heart rate within your optimal range for aerobic respiration rather than anaerobic respiration. You can find charts on the internet that will help you determine your optimal range based on your age.

Also See:
* Gluteus medius (chapter 7)
* Hamstrings (chapter 11)
* Paraspinals (chapter 3)
* Gluteus minimus (chapter 8)
* Iliopsoas (chapter 4)

You may also need to search for trigger points in the *rectus femoris*, since trigger points in this muscle can either cause similar pain referral patterns or may affect or be affected by *gluteus maximus* trigger points in some way.

Since trigger points in this muscle don't directly cause lower back and gluteal pain, it is not addressed in this book. If you can't relieve your pain with the self-help techniques in this book after six to eight weeks, you may wish to consider whether you need to treat trigger points in this additional muscle, or if you still have perpetuating factors to resolve. Go to the end of this book for other books by the author that provide self-treatment techniques of muscles not covered in this book.

Chapter 10: Piriformis

*(also Gemelli, Quadratus Femoris,
Obturator Internus, and Obturator Externus)*

Trigger points in the *piriformis* muscle are very common, and are usually involved to some extent anytime there is pain in and coming from the gluteal/pelvic region. It is commonly called "piriformis syndrome." Females are affected far more than males, with a ratio of 6:1.

When the *piriformis* muscle is enlarged, it easily entraps the sciatic nerve and other major nerves and blood vessels. Even if there is entrapment, there are also likely trigger points, which may be part of the cause of the entrapment, since trigger points may cause the muscle to bulge. Even though some or all of the sciatic nerve's fibers pass through the *piriformis* in approximately 11% of patients, Dr.'s Travell and Simons speculated that this may actually *prevent* entrapment problems, since in their research of surgeries, no surgeons had reported this nerve-muscle variation in any of their patients being operated on for sciatic nerve entrapment.

Even though the pain referral patterns of the other short lateral hip rotators (the *gemelli, quadratus femoris, obturator internus,* and *obturator externus*) have not been distinguished from those of the *piriformis*, I have had a few cases where pain was not relieved until I worked on the *obturator internus* (over the obturator foramen), so it is always worth considering that the pain may be at least partially coming from one of the other lateral rotators.

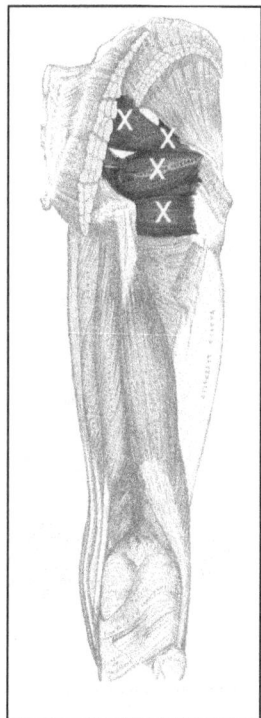

Back view, gluteal area and thigh

Common Symptoms

- referred pain primarily to the sacroiliac region (the joint where the sacrum and big pelvic bone join), over the buttock, and down the back of the thigh
- pain is worse with sitting and activity
- you may squirm a lot and shift positions trying to get comfortable, and have difficulty crossing one leg over the other knee while seated
- when lying face-up, your foot will rotate out to the side, rather than being in straight alignment
- in cases of nerve entrapment, the referred pain may extend down all the way to the calf and bottom of the foot, the gluteal muscles may atrophy, the foot may be numb and hard to walk on, and there may be swelling in the leg
- entrapment of the pudendal nerve may cause impotence in males and pain with intercourse in females, and pain in the groin or area in front of the anus

Causes and Perpetuation of Trigger Points

- reading in bed with your knees bent or otherwise sitting so that the majority of your weight is on your buttocks
- sitting on the floor, especially with your knees bent up in front of you
- sitting on your foot
- catching yourself from falling, or other sudden muscle overload
- twisting sideways while bending and lifting something heavy
- forceful rotation of your body while your weight is on one leg
- twisting repeatedly while throwing something behind you
- running

- a direct blow to the muscle
- car accidents, particularly when struck from the driver's side (even for passengers)
- driving for long periods
- foot pronation (standing with more of your weight toward the outside of your foot)
- a shorter big toe and longer second toe
- one leg *anatomically* shorter than the other (this does *not* refer to the "short leg" terminology chiropractors often use to describe the effect of vertebrae being out-of-alignment)
- over-correcting an anatomically shorter leg with a lift that is too high
- chronic pelvic inflammatory disease
- in women, spreading the legs during intercourse
- infectious sacroiliitis
- arthritis of the hip joint or hip replacement surgery, although I believe usually the trigger points likely came first and were untreated for many years
- the sacroiliac joint out-of-alignment

This is a list of perpetuating factors specific only to trigger points in <u>this</u> muscle. For a full list of perpetuating factors that can cause and perpetuate trigger points anywhere in the body and which also apply to this muscle, please see "Appendix A" (found at the end of this book), since some may need to be addressed for lasting pain relief.

Helpful Hints

- I have noticed that patients who end up with hip replacements have had chronically tight *piriformis* muscles for years. I believe this jams the joint together and causes excessive wear on the ball-and-socket joint. For this reason, I recommend to patients that they not leave *piriformis* trigger points untreated, so that they don't end up needing surgical intervention.
- As noted above, far more women have *piriformis* syndrome than men. I have noticed that women often tense their butt muscles when they are holding onto a lot of anger, and these patients tend to suffer from trigger points in the piriformis. You will need to become conscious of tightening the gluteals, and consciously relaxing them repeatedly until you re-train yourself not to tense up. You will need to deal with the underlying factors causing you to hold tension in the buttocks.
- Don't read in bed, sit on the floor, or sit in any other position that puts most of your weight on your buttocks. Sit upright with a lumbar support, so that your *hamstrings* bear some of your weight.
- Avoid running, and playing tennis, soccer and volleyball until trigger points have been inactivated.
- When sleeping, place a pillow between your legs that goes all the way from the knees to the ankles. Don't bring your legs up to a 90-degree angle.
- Don't drive for long periods without breaks. Get cruise-control so you can move your legs periodically. Be sure to use a lumbar support, and try to shift more of your weight to your *hamstrings* instead of your buttocks by adjusting the seat if possible, or by sitting on a pillow.

- If you have one leg shorter than the other or a small hemipelvis (either the right or left half of the pelvis), see a specialist for compensating lifts and pads. If you have a short big toe and longer second toe, get orthotics to prevent pronation.
- The sacroiliac joint must be treated simultaneously with the *piriformis* if the joint is a factor. See a chiropractor or osteopathic physician to be evaluated for lumbar and sacroiliac joint dysfunction.
- If you are being advised to have surgery for "piriformis syndrome," be sure to try trigger point therapy and sacroiliac joint release first, as surgery is not likely needed if these are treated first.
- You may need to see a health care provider to rule out a herniated disc. Even if you do have disc problems, you will likely benefit from trigger point therapy in order to eliminate all the pain. Acupuncture works very well on herniated and bulging disks.

Self-Help Techniques

If you develop pain deep to the lower edge of the rib cage in the area of the *diaphragm* muscle after treatment of the *piriformis* and sacroiliac joint, learn to breathe properly (see chapter 4).

Applying Pressure

Paraspinal Pressure: As part of the piriformis self-treatment, work on the *paraspinal* muscles (chapter 3), because most of the time those muscles are also involved to some extent.

Piriformis Pressure: Lying face-up, use a tennis ball on the bed and search for trigger points in the buttocks area. With your legs bent, work against the edge of the sacrum (the bony triangle between the lumbar spine and the tailbone) and all the way out toward the hip joint in a line about halfway between the top of the pelvis and the bottom curve of the butt. When you are closer to the hip joint (tense your butt muscles and there will be a big dip there), drop your knee out to the side while still keeping your knees bent and you will know when you have located the piriformis if there are trigger points in it.

Stretches

Piriformis Stretch: Lie face-up and cross your left foot over the outside of your right knee. Use your left hand to pull down on the left front of your pelvis. Use your right hand to pull down on the left knee, toward the floor, to assist in a stretch. Inhale and exhale deeply, focusing on relaxing the muscle on the exhale. Repeat on the opposite side.

Belly Dancer: While standing, place your hands on your hips and rotate your hips around in as full a circle as is comfortable. Then rotate in the opposite direction.

Also See:

* Gluteus minimus (posterior portion, chapter 8)
* Pelvic floor muscles (levator ani and coccygeus, chapter 12)
* Gluteus maximus (chapter 9)
* Gluteus medius (chapter 7)

Differential Diagnosis: If you are unable to relieve your symptoms with trigger point self-help techniques, or feel pain on both sides, you will need an MRI to rule out spinal stenosis of the central canal (narrowing of the hole that the spinal cord goes through). Acupuncture can help with the pain, but will not change the spinal stenosis. Surgery may be warranted if the pain is severe enough.

   Arthritis in the sacroiliac joint, or other types of arthritis, may cause trigger points to develop in the piriformis and may need to be ruled out.

A note to therapists: as a massage therapist, I was not able to work on the medial external portion of the obturator internus (over the obturator foramen) until I moved the patient over to the edge of the table and dropped their leg over the side. I put a chair with a pillow on it under the lower leg so the leg was bent at about 90-degrees. I was then able to treat the obturator internus by pressing in at about a 45-degree angle.

Chapter 11: Hamstrings

*(Biceps Femoris, Semitendinosus,
and Semimembranosus)*

Referred pain from trigger points in the *hamstring* muscles frequently gets diagnosed by both patients and practitioners as "sciatic pain," because of the distribution pattern down the back of the leg. At least 80% of pain down the leg comes from trigger point referral, not from "pinched nerves," a herniated disc, or stenosis in a lumbar vertebra. Since "sciatica" is usually assumed to be caused by compression on a nerve, pain referrals from trigger points are probably more aptly called "pseudo-sciatica."

Back view, gluteal area and thigh

Common Symptoms

- referred pain over the back of the thigh, around the crease of the butt, over the back of the knee, and sometimes over the calf
- pain with walking, possibly even causing a limp
- pain with getting up from a chair, particularly if your legs have been crossed
- pain on the back of the thigh, knee, and crease area of the butt when sitting, due to pressure on the trigger points
- pain in the *biceps femoris* can disrupt sleep
- it may feel like the pain is only in the *quadriceps femoris* muscle (the front of the thigh) when in fact the problem is originating in the *hamstrings*, and causing trigger points to form in the *quadriceps femoris* group
- tingling and numbness when sitting in a chair that is too high
- restricted range-of-motion when bending forward to reach your toes
- in above-knee amputees, phantom limb pain may come from trigger points in the *hamstrings*, particularly if the muscle was stretched to cover the bone

Causes and Perpetuation of Trigger Points

- strain or partial tears of the *hamstrings* as a result of inadequate stretching before a sports activity
- sitting in a chair where your feet don't touch the ground (more common in shorter people)
- sitting on a ski lift without a footrest
- children sitting in a high chair without a footrest
- a small hemipelvis (either the right or left half of the pelvis)
- treatment of *quadriceps femoris* trigger points without also treating the *hamstrings*
- auto accidents regardless of the direction of impact (in about 25% of accidents)
- short upper arms in relation to torso height that cause you to shift your weight forward when sitting

This is a list of perpetuating factors specific only to trigger points in <u>this</u> muscle. For a full list of perpetuating factors that can cause and perpetuate trigger points anywhere in the body and which also apply to this muscle, please see "Appendix A" (found at the end of this book), since some may need to be addressed for lasting pain relief.

Helpful Hints

- If your chair is too high for you (you should be able to easily slip your fingers between your chair and thigh), buy or build a sloped footstool. Patio chairs can cause problems if there is a metal bar across the front and a sagging seat bottom.
- Make sure children in high-chairs have footrests, and those at school have chairs or footrests of the proper height.
- If you swim, don't use the crawl stroke too much, but instead vary it with other strokes.
- If you bicycle, be sure your seat height is high enough that your legs can straighten out as much as possible without your knees locking.
- When driving for long periods, use cruise-control and take frequent breaks.
- You may get mis-diagnosed with sciatica, since the pain from sciatica is similar to that of *hamstrings* trigger points.
- If you have pain remaining after a laminectomy, check the *hamstrings* for trigger points.
- You may need to rule out osteoarthritis of the knee.

Self-Help Techniques

Caution: *Do not apply pressure to your legs if you have varicose veins in the area to be treated—it could release a clot that could go to your heart or brain! An acupuncturist or massage therapist should treat your legs, because they can avoid varicose veins.* However, you may still do the stretches and exercises below.

You may need to treat the *paraspinals* (chapter 3), *gluteus maximus* (chapter 9), *gluteus medius* (chapter 7), *gluteus minimus* (chapter 8) and/or *piriformis* (chapter 10) first, since these muscles can restrict range of motion, can have similar referral patterns, and/or keep *hamstrings* trigger points activated.

Applying Pressure

Hamstrings Pressure: Sit on a surface where your legs can dangle but are fully supported along the length of the thigh. Place a tennis ball under one thigh and use your hand to move the ball around to treat tender points. Repeat on the opposite thigh.

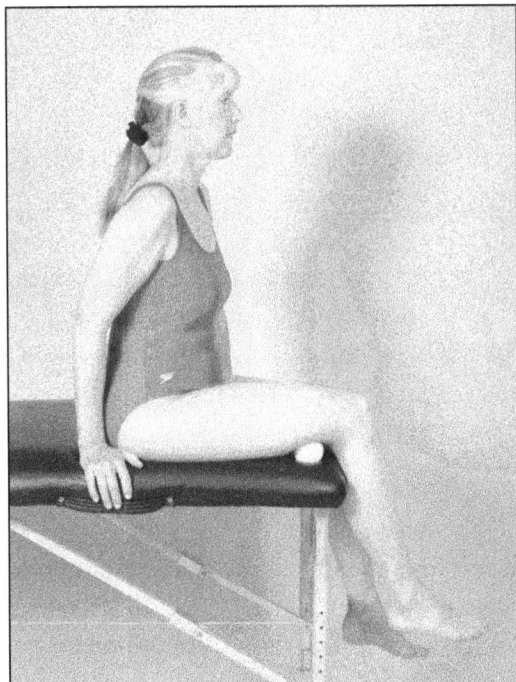

You may also treat the inner-thigh *hamstrings* by using your opposite hand to pinch the muscles between your thumb and fingers.

Stretches

In-Bathtub Stretch: See chapter 3.

Exercises

You may need to condition the *gluteus maximus* (chapter 9) in order to inactivate *hamstring* trigger points. To condition the *gluteus maximus*, you must swim, hike uphill (this muscle is minimally used for normal walking), jump, or do some other vigorous activity while keeping your heart rate within your optimal range for aerobic respiration.

Also See:

* Piriformis (piriformis and obturator internus, chapter 10)
* Gluteus medius (chapter 7)
* Gluteus minimus (posterior portion, chapter 8)
* Iliopsoas (chapter 4)

Tight *hamstrings* will tend to cause a flattened lumbar spine and a head-forward posture, resulting in problems in the *quadratus lumborum* (chapter 6), *paraspinals* (chapter 3), *iliopsoas* (chapter 4), and *rectus abdominis* (chapter 5). You should check these muscles for trigger points, particularly if you have upper-body symptoms that are only temporarily relieved. See chapter 3 for more information on head-forward posture.

You may also need to search for trigger points in the *posterior neck*, *pectoralis minor*, *infraspinatus*, *subscapularis*, *teres minor*, and *supraspinatus* muscles, since tight *hamstrings* also affect these muscles. You may also need to search for trigger points in the *popliteus*, *gastrocnemius*, *vastus lateralis*, *adductor magnus*, and *plantaris*, since trigger points in those muscles can either cause similar pain referral patterns or may affect or be affected by *hamstrings* trigger points in some way.

Since trigger points in these muscles don't directly cause lower back and gluteal pain, they are not addressed in this book. If you can't relieve your pain with the self-help techniques in this book after six to eight weeks, you may wish to consider whether you need to treat trigger points in these additional muscles, or if you still have perpetuating factors to resolve. Go to the end of this book for other books by the author that provide self-treatment techniques of muscles not covered in this book.

Differential Diagnosis: If you are unable to relieve your symptoms with trigger point self-help techniques, you may need to see a health care provider to rule out osteoarthritis of the knee. Misalignment of the sacroiliac joint and L_4 to L_5 and L_5 to S_1 vertebrae can cause spasm and restriction of the hamstring muscles. See a chiropractor or osteopathic physician for evaluation and treatment.

Chapter 12: Pelvic Floor

*(Sphincter Ani, Transverse Perinei, Levator Ani,
Coccygeus, Ischiocavernosus, Bulbospongiosus, Obturator Internus)*

Though there is little you can do for self-help for the *pelvic floor* muscles for application of pressure to trigger points, because the symptoms can be so distressing and so poorly diagnosed in relation to trigger points, I am including a chapter so you can find a professional (most likely a physical therapist trained in intra-pelvic trigger points) that can evaluate the presence of trigger points and their perpetuating factors. Women are far more affected than men -- in a group of 100 patients, 83% will be women.

Common Symptoms

Sphincter Ani
- it's hard for the patient to explain exactly where the pain is, and usually describe it as tailbone, hip, or back pain
- the area of referred pain includes the tailbone and often includes the anal area and the lower part of the sacrum (the triangular bone between the lumbar vertebrae and the tailbone)
- possibly painful bowel movements

Transverse Perinei
- it's hard for the patient to explain exactly where the pain is, and usually describe it as tailbone, hip, or back pain
- the area of referred pain includes the tailbone and often includes the anal area and the lower part of the sacrum (the triangular bone between the lumbar vertebrae and the tailbone)

Levator Ani (includes the pubococcygeus and iliococcygeus muscles)

- it's hard for the patient to explain exactly where the pain is, and usually describe it as tailbone, hip, or back pain
- the area of referred pain includes the tailbone and often includes the anal area and the lower part of the sacrum (the triangular bone between the lumbar vertebrae and the tailbone)
- trigger points may cause vaginal pain, especially during intercourse
- trigger points may cause rectal pain or pain inside the pelvis
- sitting may be uncomfortable, and pain may be aggravated by lying on the back and by bowel movements
- there may possibly be a relationship with constipation or frequent bowel movements
- pain may be diagnosed as "coccygodynia," although the tailbone itself is usually normal and not tender
- pain may also be diagnosed as "levator ani syndrome" or other similar terms

Coccygeus

- it's hard for the patient to explain exactly where the pain is, and usually describe it as tailbone, hip, or back pain
- the area of referred pain includes the tailbone and often includes the anal area and the lower part of the sacrum (the triangular bone between the lumbar vertebrae and the tailbone)
- pain may be diagnosed as "coccygodynia," although the tailbone itself is usually normal and not tender
- sitting may be painful
- trigger points are likely to a cause myofascial backache late in pregnancy and early on in labor

Ischiocavernosus

- trigger points are likely to refer pain to the genital area, such as the vagina and the base of the penis beneath the scrotum
- referred pain in the area between the scrotum or vagina and the anus

Bulbospongiosus

- trigger points are likely to refer pain to the genital area, such as the vagina and the base of the penis beneath the scrotum
- in women, possibly pain with intercourse, particularly during entry
- in women, possibly aching pain in the area between the vagina and the anus
- in men, possibly pain in the region of the backside of the scrotum, discomfort sitting erect, and sometimes a degree of impotence

Obturator Internus (intrapelvic portion)

- trigger points may cause vaginal pain
- pain may be referred to the anal and tailbone areas, and to the upper back of the thigh
- there may be referred pain and a feeling of fullness in the rectum

Post-surgical Vaginal Wall Trigger Points

- after a hysterectomy, trigger points may form in the vaginal wall which can refer pain to the lower abdomen and uterine paracervical area
- the patient usually describes the pain in what is familiar terms to them: "ovarian pain," "menstrual cramps," or "bladder spasms," and pressure on the vaginal trigger points reproduces the symptoms

Referred pain from
- sphincter ani
- levator ani
- coccygeus

Referred pain from
- obturator internus

Causes and Perpetuation of Trigger Points

- Muscle spasm and tenderness can be caused by articular dysfunction at the sacroiliac junction (the slightly moveable joint where the sacrum and the big pelvic bone meets isn't moving properly). Also, trigger points in the *pelvic floor* muscles that attach to the sacrum can destabilize the sacroiliac joint.
- Trigger points in the pelvic region can be activated by a severe fall, an auto accident, or surgery in the pelvic region.
- Most of the time it is impossible for the patient to identify a particular event that triggered the pain. In these cases, nutritional or other systemic perpetuating factors need to be identified and addressed; see "Appendix A" at the end of this book.
- *Levator ani* trigger points can be activated by sitting with a slumped posture for long periods.
- Chronic inflammation such as hemorrhoids, endometriosis, chronic salpingo-oophoritis, chronic prostatovesiculitis, and interstitial cystitis have been associated with *levator ani* spasm syndrome.

This is a list of perpetuating factors specific only to trigger points in these muscles. For a full list of perpetuating factors that can cause and perpetuate trigger points anywhere in the body and which also apply to these muscles, please see "Appendix A" (found at the end of this book), since some may need to be addressed for lasting pain relief.

Helpful Hints

- Sit upright with proper lumbar support.
- See a health care provider to identify and treat any chronic inflammations such as hemorrhoids, endometriosis, chronic salpingo-oophoritis, chronic prostatovesiculitis, and interstitial cystitis.
- See a chiropractor or osteopathic physician to identify and treat dysfunctions of the lumbrosacral, sacroiliac, and sacrococcygeal joints.
- Some physical therapists specialize in treating *pelvic* muscles, and use a variety of techniques including strengthening programs.

Treatment Techniques (for Practitioners)

Applying Pressure

The coccygeal region and the *coccygeus* muscle are more difficult to palpate from the vagina than the rectum because of the two layers of rectal mucosa and one layer of vaginal mucosa. For this reason, *a good exam and treatment must include both rectal and vaginal exams.*

The *sphincter ani, levator ani, coccygeus, obturator internus,* and *sacrococcygeus ventralis* muscles are best examined and treated through the rectum. First check for hemorrhoids, since they can make examination painful and be a cause of trigger points. If the anal sphincter has trigger points, this can also cause a great deal of pain, so the solution is to have the patient bear down to enhance relaxation as the practitioner slowly inserts a finger. If this is still too painful, try a vaginal exam.

In women, the *bulbospongiosus* muscle can only be examined vaginally. Parts of the *coccygeus* and *obturator internus* can be better examined vaginally. *The transversus perinei, ischiocavernosus,* and *bulbospongiosus* are examined externally in men, and the first two examined externally in women.

A detailed explanation of the examination of *pelvic floor* muscles is found in *Myofascial Pain and Dysfunction: The Trigger Point Manual, Vol. 2, The Lower Extremities* (Travell and Simons 1992, pp. 110–29).

Also See:

* Gluteus maximus (chapter 9)
* Piriformis (chapter 10)

APPENDIX A

What Causes and Keeps Trigger Points Going: Perpetuating Factors

> "If we treat myofascial pain syndromes without . . . correcting the multiple perpetuating factors, the patient is doomed to endless cycles of treatment and relapse. [Perpetuating factors are] the most neglected part of the management of myofascial pain syndromes . . . The answer to the question, 'How long will the beneficial results of specific myofascial therapy last?', depends largely on what perpetuating factors remain unresolved . . . One may view perpetuating factors also as predisposing factors, since their presence tends to make the muscles more susceptible to the activation of [trigger points] . . . Usually, one stress activates the [trigger point], then other factors perpetuate it. In some patients, these perpetuating factors are so important that their elimination results in complete relief of the pain without any local treatment."   ~~ *Doctors Janet Travell and David G. Simons*

There is much more to "Neuromuscular Therapy" or "Trigger Point Therapy" than learning referral patterns and how to search for trigger points; it is very important for a health care provider to identify and figure out *with* the patient what is causing and perpetuating their symptoms. This requires getting a complete medical history and evaluating for any potential perpetuating factors.

Trigger points are a *symptom*, not a *cause*. Needling or applying pressure to the trigger points treats the acute part of the problem, but does not resolve the underlying factors. If you get temporary relief from trigger point therapy but symptoms quickly recur, then trigger points are definitely a factor, but perpetuating factors need to be addressed in order to gain lasting relief.

This appendix will outline some general causes of trigger point activation and how to address the factors, and each muscle chapter will specifically address issues particularly pertinent to that muscle. I recommend you read all of the perpetuating factors, since you likely have more than one factor that you may not have recognized up to this point.

Acute or Chronic Viral, Bacterial, and Parasitic Infections

Acute infections, such as **colds, flu, strep throat, and bronchitis** will aggravate trigger points, particularly in a person with fibromyalgia or chronic fatigue. It is important to head off illness at the first sign in order to avoid perpetuating trigger points. When you start to get sick, take the Chinese herbs Gan Mao Ling or Yin Chiao, Echinacea, and/or homeopathics such as Osillococcinum or other appropriate homeopathics for colds, flu, or sinusitis. Once you are past the initial stage of illness, if symptoms progress, the Chinese herbs you take will be determined by your particular set of symptoms, so at this point you may need professional help to determine the proper herbs. You should have the above-mentioned herbs and homeopathics available at home so you can treat your symptoms as soon as you notice the first signs. This is particularly important if you have fibromyalgia, sinusitis, asthma, or other recurrent infections, since your trigger points will be activated by illness, and getting sick can set you back by weeks in your treatment and healing.

Outbreaks of **chronic infections**, such as **herpes simplex** (cold sores, genital herpes, herpes zoster) will also aggravate trigger points, and may need to be managed if recurrence is frequent. There are many pharmaceutical drugs and natural supplements/herbs for treating recurrent herpes infections, and some will work better than others for you. Also, if you are getting recurrent outbreaks you will want figure out what is stressing your immune system, such as allergies or emotional stress. Sometimes a herpes outbreak is the first sign you are fighting an acute illness, so that is the time to take the above-mentioned supplements.

Other chronic infections such as **sinus infections, an abscessed or impacted tooth, or urinary tract infections** will perpetuate trigger points. If you suspect a **tooth**, you will need to see your dentist for evaluation. **Urinary tract infections** (UTI's) need to be dealt with promptly. You may use over-the-counter western drugs, Chinese herbs, and cranberry (don't use sweetened juice), but if you don't respond to treatment immediately you will need to see your health care provider, since UTI's can turn into life-threatening kidney infections. Any mechanical reasons for **sinus infections** need to be dealt with for lasting relief. Naturopathic doctors can use a small inflatable balloon to open up the passages. You may need surgical intervention if the blockage is severe enough. Many people report success using a Neti Pot (get it at your health food store) to flush the sinuses with a warm saline solution. With both sinus infections and UTI's, antibiotics often won't kill all of the pathogens, and you may get a lingering, recurrent infection. However, antibiotics also work quickly, so I often recommend to patients that they combine antibiotics, acupuncture, herbs, and homeopathics to knock the infection out as quickly and completely as possible so it doesn't become a chronic problem.

The fish tapeworm, giardia, and occasionally amoeba are the most likely **parasites** to perpetuate trigger points. The fish tapeworm and giardia scar the lining of the intestine and impair your ability to absorb nutrients, and they also consume vitamin B-12. **Amoeba** can produce toxins that are passed from the intestine into the body. **Fish tapeworms** can be transmitted from raw fish. **Giardia** is most often associated with drinking untreated water from streams, but it can also be passed by an infected person not washing their hands after a bowel movement, particularly if they are preparing food or have some other hand-to-mouth contact.

Any time you have **chronic diarrhea** it is worth testing for parasites. A cheaper alternative is just to treat with herbs like grapefruit seed extract or Pulsatilla (a Chinese herb) and see if your symptoms improve. Since these will also kill off the good intestinal flora, you will want to follow treatment with a good multi-acidophilus supplement, as you would after any antibiotic. If you have blood in your stools, you should always see your health care provider immediately to rule out serious conditions. Acupuncture and Naturopathy can help resolve chronic diarrhea from most causes.

There is substantial controversy about whether **systemic candida infections** exist, though it is now listed in the Merck Manual (a medical text of illness and disease). There is abundant information on the Web regarding this subject, so I won't go into detail. Candida is a normal intestinal flora, but can multiply beyond a normal amount and cause a variety of symptoms including muscular pain. Many people report feeling much better on an anti-candida diet, and in any case it is a pretty healthy way to eat. There are many herbal products on the market for eliminating candida, including grapefruit seed extract, oil of oregano, Echinacea, Pulsatilla, and many formulas. Again, you will want to follow any of these with a good multi-acidophilus supplement to replace the beneficial intestinal flora.

Allergies and other Environmental Stressors

Both inhaled and ingested allergens perpetuate trigger points and make them harder to treat due to the subsequent histamine release. Skin tests are useful for testing for **inhaled allergens**, and there are a few methods for testing for **food allergens**.

One of the best ways to test for **food allergens** is an elimination diet, where you eliminate all foods, add them back in one at a time, and then rotate foods. You can find instructions for this in *"Prescription for Nutritional Healing"* by Balch and Balch under "Allergies." The challenge with a rotation diet is that most people are not willing to do it, as it takes a very strict control of your diet and a careful food diary for a month. As an alternative, Balch and Balch offer a quick-test. After sitting and relaxing for a few minutes, take your pulse rate for one minute, then eat the food you are testing. Keep still for 15-20 minutes and take your pulse again. If your pulse rate has increased more than ten beats per minute, eliminate this food from your diet for one month, then re-test. Naturopathic doctors offer a blood test for food sensitivities. Food allergens and sensitivities must be eliminated, but this can become challenging when you eat at other people's homes, when dining out, or while traveling. Try to keep something you *can* have with you, so you have an alternative.

There may be some ingested substances to which you are not allergic, but can aggravate your condition anyway and should be avoided. Chinese diagnosis differentiates pain by the quality of the pain (dull, achy, sharp, shooting, stabbing, burning, moving) and what makes it better or worse (i.e., rest/activity, heat/cold/damp, etc.), and some foods will aggravate certain conditions. You can see an Oriental Medicine practitioner for an evaluation of your pain and to get dietary advice, but you can try eliminating the following foods to see if it helps: coffee and black tea (yes, even decaf!), alcohol, bananas, peanuts, dairy, greasy foods, pop, sugar, wheat, and spicy foods.

Environmental allergies must be controlled as much as possible, and if you see a specialist for a skin test to identify allergens, they will make specific suggestions based on the allergen. A good HEPA air filter will help substantially, and you will need one for each room. Make sure each unit is large enough to cover the needed square footage. Not all air filters are equal, so be sure to research your options. An ozonator will kill molds, but I do not suggest leaving one running while you or pets are in the room, even though some are made for that purpose. Get an ozonator that puts out enough ozone that you can "bomb" the room while you and your pets are gone. Bomb one room at a time and close the door so that you will get a high concentration. After a few hours, hold your breath and open the windows and let the room air out for a couple of minutes before you occupy the room again. You will smell ozone (like lightening) lingering, but the air is fine to breathe after just a few minutes, so don't be concerned.

Seasonal Affective Disorder (SAD) affects millions of people to one degree or another, particularly people living closer to the North or South poles where the daylight hours are shorter in winter. SAD causes symptoms such as depression, loss of energy, decreased activity, fatigue, sleeping up to four extra hours per night, irritability and crying spells, difficulty concentrating, carbohydrate cravings, and increased appetite and weight gain. Though SAD probably does not directly cause pain, many of these symptoms *can* contribute to pain eventually. For example, if increased activity helps reduce your pain but SAD keeps you from exercising, then the SAD needs to be treated in order to help reduce your pain. Most SAD patients improve when they get additional light in their retinas. Unless you sit right next to a window in your office, you are probably not getting enough light. You may be traveling to and from work in the dark much of the year. One solution is to make sure you get outside during daylight hours, possibly for a walk at your lunch hour. Another solution is to buy a therapeutic light box. Full-spectrum lights alone are not strong enough to be of therapeutic value, so you need to get a box with reflective materials capable of producing 10,000 LUX. You need to be within 24" of the box in most cases (the light box should come with instructions that tell you how close you need to be to get 10,000 LUX), and you need to have your eyes open and looking toward the box so you get the light in your retinas.

      Toxic metals exposure has been implicated in pain syndromes. A hair analysis obtained through a naturopathic doctor can evaluate toxic levels of chemicals and mineral levels. If you find you have high levels of toxic metals, the doctor can help you with a detox program.

Emotional Factors

      While it is important to recognize the role of stress and emotional factors in creating and perpetuating illness, unfortunately all too often patients are dismissed (or medicated) by their health care providers as "just being under stress." They depart the health care provider's office with their physical symptoms not being assessed or addressed, particularly when it comes to the symptoms of pain and depression. This seems to happen more frequently to women, but I've also had male patients who had the same experience.

      Antidepressants are often prescribed, which may possibly help with the acute symptoms, but the side-effects can add to the underlying condition causing the symptoms, and a vicious cycle ensues. If you are in pain long enough, of *course* you will begin to get fatigued and depressed. If you are depressed long enough, you will probably develop pain. Anything that has gone on long enough *will* have both components.

      One of the things I like most about Oriental Medicine and homeopathy is that both modalities assume you cannot separate the physical body from the emotions, and symptoms of both are used to develop a diagnosis, and are treated simultaneously. With acupuncture there are no side-effects, and response is usually rapid. With both homeopathy and herbs (Chinese or American) the wrong prescription or dosage can have side-effects, just as with Western prescription drugs, so it is important to consult with a trained professional.

      If you are **angry, anxious or stressed**, chances are you are holding at least some of your body parts very tense, and developing trigger points. You may be hiking your shoulders up around your neck, tightening your forearms or abdomen, or tensing your gluteal muscles (women tense their gluteal muscles more often than men). In addition to dealing with the underlying cause of emotional factors, you will have to notice when you are tensing body parts, and keep consciously relaxing them over and over again. You are re-training yourself to not tense your muscles. Bio-feedback can help with this.

If you are experiencing an unusual desire to be alone, a disinterest in your favorite activities, a decrease in job performance, and are neglecting your appearance and hygiene, you may be suffering from **depression**. Other symptoms of depression are insomnia, loss of appetite, weight loss, impotence or a lowered libido, blurred vision, a sad mood, thoughts of suicide or death, an inability to concentrate, a poor memory, indecision, mumbled speech, and negative reactions to suggestions. No one symptom will confirm a diagnosis of depression, because there are other reasons for some of these symptoms. It is the combination of symptoms that confirms a depression diagnosis. Depression lowers your pain threshold, increases pain, and adversely affects your response to trigger point therapy. (See the section on Organ Dysfunction and Disease, **thyroid**, below, since thyroid problems can be an undiagnosed cause of depression.)

If you are angry, depressed, anxious, or stressed, you will need to address this in some manner in order to speed recovery from pain. Often people suffering from severe emotional factors, chronic fatigue and/or extreme pain lack the energy to participate in their own healing. You may have difficulty feeding yourself properly or even getting out of bed, and cannot manage even mild forms of exercise such as walking -- the very things that would help you start to feel better. You may have difficulty making it to your appointments. If this describes you, you will need to do *whatever you can* to get to the point where you can start taking better care of yourself. This may mean getting antidepressants, acupuncture, homeopathy, counseling, pain relievers, and/or doing the self-help techniques in this book. Walking and deep breathing are great tension and depression-relievers. Even walking ten minutes per day (especially outside) can be extremely beneficial. Just doing one of these things will help get you started in the right direction and improve your energy and outlook.

"Secondary Gains"

Sometimes we subconsciously get something out of being sick or in pain. For example, if you have a hard time saying "no," it is easier to excuse yourself by not feeling well, rather than having to bear the brunt of the reactions you get from people who aren't used to you refusing their requests or demands. Some people have a need to stay in pain in order to get attention. Perhaps in childhood that was the only way they could get their parent's attention and they are still using that strategy as an adult. Sometimes it's easier to focus on physical symptoms than deal with underlying anxiety and emotional problems. Some people have financial reasons for not getting well, such as disability payments or lawsuit settlements, or it may get them out of some things they don't want to do.

If you find yourself complaining about your physical symptoms but not doing anything to relieve them, you might want to ask yourself what you may be getting out of staying sick. This is not always the case, as in severe depression, but it is worth at least exploring. Chances are, if you have purchased this book, you do not have subconscious needs to stay sick or in pain, since you have already taken a step to help yourself.

Good Sport Syndrome

Many people believe in pushing through the pain -- that it will make them stronger and is beneficial. Wrong! This just aggravates existing problems and makes them harder to treat. Exercise should be comfortable, such as alternating running with walking or resting in between weight repetitions, and using weights that aren't too heavy. If you tend to overdo things, you will need to back off on your activities and add them back in slowly with the guidance of your practitioner. Returning to activities too soon or excessively will quickly wipe out your therapeutic progress.

Injuries

A healthy muscle is pliable to the touch when it is not being used, but will feel firm if called upon for action. If a muscle feels firm at rest, it is tight in an unhealthy way (even if you work-out). I like to use an analogy of a rubber band or stick. Imagine that a sudden, unexpected force is applied to the "stick," or tight muscle (such as a fall). Like a stick, the muscle will be damaged. If a sudden force is applied to a pliable muscle, or "rubberband," it will stretch with the force instead, and will be much less likely to be injured. Since latent trigger points restrict range-of-motion to some degree, and almost everyone has some latent trigger points, a muscle may be tight and restricted without you being aware of it, and can be easily injured if a sudden force is applied.

Injuries are one of the most common initiators of trigger points. **People who exercise regularly are less likely to develop trigger points** than those who exercise occasionally and overdo it. If you have an injury, begin treatment as soon as possible. Apply cold during the first 48 hours, and use some form of arnica homeopathic orally and/or topically as soon as possible. There are Chinese herb formulas for trauma that you can get from an acupuncturist or possibly a health food store. Have these available in your medicine cabinet since it may be hard for you to go to the store after you are injured, and because these work best when started immediately after the injury. See an acupuncturist or massage therapist who is experienced in working with recent injuries. You may also need to see a chiropractor, osteopathic physician, or physical therapist.

Surgeries will likely leave some amount of scar tissue, which can perpetuate trigger points in adjacent muscle fibers. **Scar tissue** can be broken up to an extent with cross-friction massage. Because this is usually fairly painful, I only work on scars for a few minutes each appointment, and I warn the patient that it will be painful but that I won't do it for more than a few minutes. Most patients will not work on their own scars vigorously enough due to the pain level. Acupuncture can treat scar tissue and help eliminate the pain from trigger points around the area. I recommend using both cross-friction massage and acupuncture as part of the treatment protocol, rather than just one or the other.

Mechanical Stresses

Chronic mechanical stresses are one of the most common causes of trigger point activation and perpetuation, and are nearly always correctable. A **skeletal asymmetry**, including an anatomically shorter leg and a small hemipelvis (either the right or left half of the pelvis) can be corrected with shoe lifts and butt lifts. [NOTE: In this book, reference to a "shorter leg" refers to a *true* anatomical leg length inequality where the bones are shorter on one side, rather than the "shorter leg" caused by a spinal mis-alignment, which is a term chiropractors use.] A **skeletal disproportion**, such as a long second toe can be corrected with shoe orthotics, and short upper arms can be corrected with ergonomically correct furniture. Vertebral subluxation and other bones-out-alignment can be adjusted by a chiropractor or osteopathic physician, especially if the muscles are also first relaxed by an acupuncturist or massage therapist. Your physical therapist may be trained in manipulations.

Wearing appropriate shoes can help relieve symptoms in your entire body (see "Abuse of Muscles," below). **Orthotics** can help even more. My favorite non-corrective orthotics are the Superfeet brand. They have a deep heel cup which helps prevent pronation (more weight on the inside of your foot) and supination (more weight on the outside of the foot), and they have excellent arch support. Superfeet has a variety of models, including cheaper non-custom "Trim-to-Fit" footbeds, and moderately-priced custom molded footbeds to provide support in a variety of footwear. See Superfeet.com to learn more about their products. If you find you need corrective orthotics, you will need to see a podiatrist. If you decide to get custom orthotics, be sure to work on your trigger points first, because as the muscles relax you will stand differently and the orthotics need to be formed for the corrected stance.

Misfitting furniture is a major cause of muscular pain, particularly in the work place. There are companies that specialize in coming into your work place and correcting your office arrangement, and fitting you for furniture that fits your body. Your employer may balk at the cost, but if they don't change your misfitting furniture, they will end up paying for it in lost work time and worker's compensation claims.

I see a lot of what I call "mouse injuries" -- arm and shoulder pain due to using a computer mouse for extended periods of time without proper arm support. The keyboard should be kept as close to lap level as possible. When not using your computer, your elbows and forearms should rest evenly on either your work surface or armrests of the proper height. Your computer screen should be directly in front of you with the middle of the screen slightly below eye level, and the copy attached to the side of the screen, so that you may look directly forward as much as possible. Your knees should fit under your desk, and the chair needs to be close enough that you can lean against your backrest. A good chair will have a backrest with a slope of 25 to 30-degrees back from the vertical which supports both the lumbar area and the mid-back. The seat should be low enough that your feet rest flat on the floor without compression of the thigh by the front edge of the seat, high enough that not all the pressure is put on the buttocks, and slightly hollowed out to accommodate the buttocks. The armrests must be high enough to provide support for the elbows without having to lean to the side, but not so high as to cause the shoulders to hike up. The upholstery needs to be firm and casters should be avoided. I highly recommend headsets for phones to solve neck and back pain.

A lumbar support helps correct round-shouldered posture. Most chiropractic offices carry lumbar supports of varying thickness. I recommend getting one for the car (most car seats actually *curve the wrong way* in the lumbar area) and your favorite seat at home, and investing in a good chair for the office, even if your employer won't. Try to avoid sitting in or on anything without back support, which causes you to sit with your shoulders and upper back slumped forward. When going to sporting events, picnics, or other places you won't have a back support, bring a *Crazy Creek Chair*™ (or something similar) to provide at least some support. You can get one through most of the major sporting goods suppliers for about $49, a good investment in your back, and they are very lightweight for carrying. Or consider a lightweight collapsible chair, also available at sporting goods stores.

Sleeping in a sagging bed can cause back and hip problems. (See the section on Sleep Problems below).

But properly fitting furniture won't help as much if you are not also conscientious of avoiding **poor posture**. If you slouch at your desk or on your couch at home, or read in bed, for example, your muscles will suffer. **Abuse of muscles** includes poor body mechanics (i.e., lifting improperly), long periods of immobility (i.e., sitting at a desk without a break), repetitive movements (i.e., computer use), holding your body in an awkward position for long periods (i.e., dentists and mechanics), and excessively quick and jerky movements (i.e., sports). Learn to lift properly and take frequent breaks from anything you must do for long time periods.

If you have a habit of immobilizing your muscles to protect against pain, you will need to start gently increasing your range of motion as you inactivate trigger points. Don't keep stressing the muscles to see if it still hurts or to demonstrate to your treating professionals where you have to move it to in order to get it to hurt -- if you keep repeating this motion, you will just keep the trigger points activated.

Be sure to sit while putting clothing on your lower body. Don't wear high heels or cowboy boots. If you carry a purse, get a strap long enough that you can wear it diagonally across your body, rather than over one shoulder. If you use a day pack, put the straps over both shoulders. Without realizing it, you are hiking up one shoulder at least a little to keep the straps from slipping off no matter *how* light your purse or pack may be. Notice whether you hold your shoulders up or are tightening muscles such as your butt, arms, or abdomen when you are under stress. You will need to re-train yourself to break this habit.

If you are clenching your jaw or grinding your teeth, see a dentist for help. The soft plastic bite splints found over-the-counter in pharmacies are too soft and do not help temporomandibular joint dysfunction. You need to be fitted by your dentist for a hard, slippery acrylic night guard.

Constricting clothing can lead to muscular problems. My rule of thumb is, if the clothing item leaves an elastic mark or indentation in the skin, it is too tight and is cutting off proper circulation. Check your bras, socks, ties, and belts to see if they are too tight.

Be sure to check muscles listed in the muscle chapters that can cause "satellite trigger points," since this is one perpetuating cause. For example, if you find trigger points in the abdominal muscles but trigger points quickly recur, check the paraspinal muscles also, because trigger points there can refer to the abdominal area and cause trigger points to be reactivated.

Nutritional Problems and Diet

Doctors Travell and Simons found that almost half of their patients required treatment for **vitamin inadequacies** to obtain lasting relief from the pain and dysfunction of trigger points, and thought it was one of the most important perpetuating factors to address. They found **the most important were the water-soluble vitamins B-1, B-6, B-12, folic acid, vitamin C, and the minerals calcium, magnesium, iron and potassium**. Other researchers have now added **vitamin D** to that list.

The more deficient in nutrients you are, the more symptoms you will have, and your trigger points and nervous system will be more hyper-irritable. Even if a blood test determines you are at the low end of the normal range, you may still need more of a nutrient, since your body will pull nutrients from the tissues before it will allow a decrease in the blood levels. Several factors may lead to nutrient insufficiency:

- An inadequate intake of a nutrient

- Impaired nutrient absorption
- Inadequate nutrient utilization
- An increased need by the body
- A nutrient leaving the body too quickly
- A nutrient being destroyed within the body too quickly

You may be in a **high risk group** if you are: elderly, pregnant or nursing, an alcoholic or other drug user, poor, depressed, or seriously ill. If you tend to diet by leaving out important food groups, or have an eating disorder, you will also deplete yourself of necessary nutrients.

- Even if you have a fairly healthy diet, because our soils have been depleted in nutrients from too frequent crop-rotations, chemical fertilizers, and long shipping distances, our food does not provide all the nutrition we require. In addition, many of us don't have a very balanced diet, and processed foods do not contain as much nutrition as fresh-prepared. Most people need to take some kind of **multi-supplement** to ensure proper nutrition, especially if you fall into one of the high risk groups mentioned above. Because some vitamins require the presence of other vitamins, a good multi-supplement ensures the needed combination is present. Be sure to check the label to make sure there are adequate minerals in a multi -- you may need to also take a multi-mineral. Improving your nutrient intake to see if it improves your symptoms is an easy and relatively inexpensive therapy to try. Take your vitamins with food, since some need to bind with substances found in food in order to be absorbed.

  Building up sufficient levels of vitamin B-12, vitamin D, and iron may take several months; don't get discouraged if you don't see immediate results, though you may start gradually feeling better within a few weeks from taking multivitamin and multimineral supplements.

- You may still need to be tested by a health care provider for inadequacies, since some people are not able to absorb certain nutrients, and need to have them injected or mega-dosed. For example, some people cannot absorb B-12, and need to get intramuscular injections to provide that necessary vitamin.

- **Take your vitamins and herbs when you are *not* sick** -- the germs also like the vitamins and herbs and they will get stronger. See the section above on Acute or Chronic Viral, Bacterial, and Parasitic Infections for suggestions on how to head off illness. Once all symptoms have abated, you may switch back to your regular vitamins and herbs.

- How well your **digestive system** is functioning is also a factor. If you are not digesting well, you do not have enough enzymes or possibly hydrochloric acid to break down food properly. Taking digestive enzymes or hydrochloric acid for long periods is not a good solution, because they will take over the natural function of your body. Supplementation can be used in the short term, but you need to repair the body's natural function so it can perform its own job properly. **Digestive problems** can be addressed with the help of an acupuncturist, herbalist, or naturopath. They can give you dietary recommendations based on your unique set of health problems and constitution, and prescribe herbs to re-balance your systems.

- It is a common mis-conception that raw foods and whole grains are the healthiest way to eat. It is actually better to **cook your food** (not overcook!) in order to start the chemical breakdown process, so your digestive system doesn't have to work as hard. If you are having trouble digesting, white rice and bread are easier to digest than whole grains. Soups are nutritious and easy to digest.

- **Fasting** is hard on the digestive system. If you want to do a cleanse, use herbs and psyllium, but don't stop eating.

- Most people should not be strict vegetarians. At the very least you should eat organic eggs for a **high-quality protein** source. Most vegetarians are not very good about combining foods, and even if they are, most still seem to feel better when they add high-quality animal protein back into their diet. Plant sources contain mainly the pyridoxol form of B-6, but animal sources contain both the pyridoxal and pyridoxamine forms of B-6, and are less susceptible to the loss of the vitamin due to cooking or preserving. B-12 is *only* found in animal proteins, including dairy products. Brewer's yeast does not contain B-12, unless the yeast is grown on a special B-12-containing substrate.

- If you have **chronic diarrhea**, you will not retain food long enough in the intestines to absorb nutrients. You will need to identify and eliminate the source of diarrhea. Acupuncture, herbs, and dietary changes can often successfully address this problem.

- Excess **caffeine** increases muscle tension and trigger point irritability, leading to increased pain. Dr.'s Travell and Simons state that "... caffeine has long been known to cause a persistent contracture, or caffeine rigor, of muscle fibers. This rigor is due to enhancement by caffeine of the release of calcium from the sarcoplasmic reticulum and to interference with the rebinding of calcium ions by the sarcoplasmic reticulum." They found that caffeine in excess of 150 mg daily (more than two eight-ounce cups of regular coffee) would lead to caffeine rigor. Based on my clinical experience, some people can't even consume 150 mg without aggravating their pain. In counting your daily intake, be sure to count any caffeine in the drugs you are taking, and remember that espresso and similar drinks will have far greater amounts of caffeine. There are websites that list caffeine amounts for foods and beverages.

- **Alcohol** aggravates trigger points by decreasing serum and tissue folate levels. It increases the body's need for vitamin C, while decreasing the body's ability to absorb it. **Tobacco** also increases the need for vitamin C. In Chinese Medicine, caffeine and alcohol are said to be very "qi stagnating." **Marijuana** is very stagnating also, and stays in your system for about three months after smoking it. Stagnation is one cause of pain, therefore using any of the above substances will increase your pain level.

- Eliminating foods and beverages that aggravate your condition (such as allergins, coffee, and alcohol) may not be enough, if the underlying condition that was caused by the food has not been resolved. For example, if you have been eating damp-producing foods (like dairy and peanut butter) which has led to dampness in the muscles (as in fibromyalgia), even if you stop ingesting the food or beverage you still have dampness in the muscles that must be eliminated. Plan on avoiding the necessary foods for two months minimum *in conjunction* with acupuncture and/or herbs and other supplements, in order to determine whether eliminating the food is helpful. Many people will stop ingesting a food or drink for one week, decide it hasn't made a difference, and then re-start their regular diet. Or the food or beverage is so important to them that they'd rather have pain and other medical conditions, than give the substance up. Reaching a conclusion after one week is one way to justify continuing to ingest the substance.

- **Herbs** should be taken with the advice of a qualified practitioner. I've seen many people who have injured their digestive systems by taking too many herbs, or herbs that are improper for their conditions and constitution. What may be the correct herb for a friend or a family member may not be the correct herb for you, so seek professional advice.

- Room-temperature **water** is better than cold drinks -- if you drink something cold, your stomach has to work harder to warm it up, and it taxes the digestive system. Drink about two quarts per day, or more if you have a larger body mass or sweat a lot. A general rule of thumb for kids and adults weighing more than 100 pounds is your body weight multiplied by the number of ounces (i.e., 140 lbs. = 70 ounces). Drink at least one extra quart per day if it is very hot out, and extra water during and immediately after a work-out. If you drink *too* much water, you can deplete Vitamin B-1 (thiamine). Thirst is not necessarily a good indicator of whether or not you are dehydrated. Your urine should be a light yellow, unless you have just taken a multivitamin or B-vitamin supplement.

- **Don't drink distilled water**, because you need the minerals found in non-distilled water. If you drink bottled water, make sure you know its source, and that it is not distilled. This industry is not currently regulated, so you may need to do some research on the company.

Vitamins

- **Vitamin C** reduces post-exercise soreness and corrects the capillary fragility which leads to easy bruising. (Hint: if you don't remember how you got a bruise, you are likely bruising too easily.) It is essential for collagen formation (connective tissue) and forming bones. Vitamin C is required for synthesis of the neurotransmitters norepinephrine and serotonin, is needed for your body's response to stress, is important for immune system function, and decreases the irritability of trigger points caused by infection.

Too *much* Vitamin C can lead to watery diarrhea or non-specific urethritis. However, Vitamin C helps terminate diarrhea due to food allergies. Vitamin C daily doses above 400mg are not used by the body, and 1000mg/day increases the risk of kidney stone formation, so mega-dosing with Vitamin C is not necessary nor recommended. Women taking estrogen or oral contraceptives may need 500mg/day.

Vitamin C is likely to be deficient in smokers, alcoholics, older people (the presence of Vitamin C in the tissues decreases with age), infants fed primarily on cows' milk (usually between the ages of 6-12 months), people with chronic diarrhea, psychiatric patients, and fad dieters. Initial symptoms of deficiency include weakness, lethargy, irritability, vague aching pains in the joints and muscles, easy bruising, and possibly weight loss. In severe cases of Vitamin C deficiency (scurvy), the gums become red, swollen, bleed easily, and teeth may become loose and fall out.

Do not take Vitamin C with antacids; since Vitamin C is ascorbic acid, and the purpose of an antacid is to neutralize acid, antacids will neutralize Vitamin C and make it ineffective. Food sources include citrus fruits and *fresh* juices, *raw* broccoli, *raw* Brussels sprouts, collard, kale, turnip greens, guava, *raw* sweet peppers, cabbage, and potatoes

- **Taking too many vitamins A, D, and E, and folic acid** can cause symptoms similar to deficiencies, so don't mega-dose on those supplements unless a health care provider has determined your condition warrants it.

- **Thiamine (Vitamin B-1)** is essential for normal nerve function and energy production within muscle cells. Diminished pain and temperature sensitivity and an inability to detect vibrations indicate you are low in thiamine. You may also possibly experience calf cramping at night, slight sweating, constipation, and fatigue. B-1 is needed for proper thyroid hormone levels (see the section on Organ Dysfunction and Disease below). Abuse of alcohol reduces thiamine absorption, and absorption is further reduced if liver disease is also present. The tannin in black tea, antacid use, and a magnesium deficiency can also prevent the absorption of thiamine. Thiamine can be destroyed by processing foods, and by heating them to temperatures above 212º F (100º C). Thiamine is excreted too rapidly when taking diuretics or drinking too much water. Lean pork, kidney, liver, beef, eggs, fish, beans, nuts, and some whole grain cereals (if the hull and germ are present) are good sources of thiamine.

- **Pyridoxine (Vitamin B-6)** is important for nerve function, energy metabolism, amino acid metabolism, and synthesis of neurotransmitters including norepinephrine and serotonin, which strongly influence pain perception. Deficiency of B-6 results in anemia, reduced absorption and storage of B-12, increased excretion of Vitamin C, blocked synthesis of niacin, and can lead to a hormonal imbalance. Deficiency of B-6 will manifest as symptoms of one of the other B-vitamins, since B-6 is needed in order for all the others to perform their functions. The need for B-6 increases with age and increased protein consumption. Tropical sprue and alcohol use interfere with its absorption. Use of **oral contraceptives** increases your requirement for B-6, and impairs glucose tolerance. This can lead to depression if you don't supplement with B-6, particularly if you already have a history of depression. Corticosteroid use, excessive alcohol use, pregnancy and lactation, antitubercular drugs, uremia, and hyperthyroidism also increase the need for B-6. Sources of B-6 include liver, kidney, chicken (white meat), halibut, tuna, English walnuts, soybean flour, navy beans, bananas, and avocados. There is also some amount of B-6 present in yeast, lean beef, egg yolk, and whole wheat.

- **Cobalamin (Vitamin B-12) and Folic Acid** need to be taken together to form erythrocytes (a type of red blood cell) and rapidly dividing cells such as those found in the gastrointestinal tract, and for fatty acid synthesis used in the formation of parts of certain nerve fibers. B-12 is needed for both fat and carbohydrate metabolism. A deficiency can result in **pernicious (megaloblastic) anemia**, which reduces oxygen coming to the site of the trigger point, adding to the dysfunctional cycle and increasing pain. A deficiency of B-12 may also cause symptoms such as non-specific depression, fatigue, an exaggerated startle reaction to noise or touch, and an increased susceptibility to trigger points. B-12 is only found in animal products or supplements. Several drugs may impair the absorption of B-12, as can mega-doses of Vitamin C for long periods of time.

- A **folate deficiency** (also known as **folic acid** when in the synthetic form) can cause you to be fatigued easily, sleep poorly, and feel discouraged and depressed. It can cause "restless legs," diffuse muscular pain, diarrhea, a loss of sensation in the extremities, and you may feel cold frequently, along with a slightly lower basal body temperature than the "normal" 98.6º F (37º C). Folic acid deficiency is very prevalent and can lead to **megaloblastic anemia**. In the U.S., studies have shown that at least 15% of Caucasians are deficient, while at least 30% of African-Americans and Latinos are deficient. At least half of Canadians eat less than the dietary recommendation. Part of the problem is that 50-95% of the folate content of foods may be destroyed in food processing and preparation, so even if you eat folate sources, you may not be receiving the benefit. A necessary conversion in the digestive system is inhibited by peas, beans, citrus fruits, acidic foods, and antacids, so eat these separately from your folic acid sources. The best sources of folate are leafy vegetables, yeast, organ meat, fruit, and lightly cooked vegetables such as broccoli and asparagus. You are at greatest risk for folate deficiency if you are elderly, have a bowel disorder, are pregnant or lactating, or use drugs and alcohol regularly. Certain other drugs will also deplete folate, such as anti-inflammatories (including aspirin), diuretics, estrogens (such as birth control pills), and anti-convulsants. You must also have adequate B-12 intake in order to absorb folic acid, plus only taking one of these can mask a severe deficiency in the other.

- **Vitamin D** is required for both the absorption and the utilization of calcium and phosphorus. It is necessary for growth and thyroid function, it protects against muscle weakness, and helps regulate the heartbeat. It is important for the prevention of cancer, osteoarthritis, osteoporosis, and calcium deficiency. A mild deficiency of vitamin D may manifest as a loss of appetite, a burning sensation in the mouth and throat, diarrhea, insomnia, visual problems, and weight loss. It has been estimated that close to 90% of patients with chronic musculoskeletal pain may have a vitamin D deficiency.

Vitamin D-3 is synthesized by the skin when exposed to the sun's UV rays. Unfortunately, many people don't get enough sun exposure, especially if they live at latitudes or in climates with little sun available during the winter months. Exposing your face and arms to the sun for 15 minutes three times per week will ensure that your body synthesizes an adequate amount of vitamin D. Because the amount of exposure needed varies from person to person and also depends on geographical location, you will need to do some personal research and perhaps consult with a dermatologist to determine the proper amount for you. Food sources of vitamin D include salmon, halibut, sardines, tuna, and eggs. Other sources include dairy products, dandelion greens, liver, oatmeal, and sweet potatoes. If you take supplements, look for the D-3 form, or fish oil capsules.

Minerals

Inadequate salt, calcium/magnesium, or potassium can lead to **muscle cramping**.

- Do not entirely eliminate **salt** from your diet, especially if you sweat. You do need some salt in your diet (unless you have been instructed otherwise by your health care provider for certain medical conditions), though you don't want to overdo it either.

- **Calcium, magnesium, potassium, and iron** are needed for proper muscle function. Iron is required for oxygen transport to the muscle fibers. Calcium is essential for releasing acetylcholine at the nerve terminal, and both calcium and magnesium are needed for the contracting mechanism of the muscle fiber. Potassium is needed to get the muscle fiber quickly ready for its next contraction. Deficiency of these minerals increases the irritability of trigger points. Calcium, magnesium, and potassium should be taken together, because an increase in one can deplete the others. Also needed for good health but not as important for muscle function are zinc, iodine, copper, manganese, chromium, selenium, and molybdenum.

  It is especially important to take **calcium** for at least a few years prior to menopause to help prevent osteoporosis. Vitamin D is needed for calcium uptake. Food sources of calcium include dairy (though this is not recommended for people with damp conditions, such as fibromyalgia), salmon, sardines, seafood, green leafy vegetables, almonds, asparagus, blackstrap molasses, brewer's yeast, broccoli, cabbage, carob, collards, dandelion greens, figs, filberts, kale, kelp, mustard greens, oats, parsley, prunes, sesame seeds, tofu, turnip greens, and whey.

- Do not take Tums or other **antacids** as a source of **calcium**. Stomach acid is needed for the uptake of calcium, but an antacid neutralizes stomach acid. So even if there is calcium present, it cannot be used. If you must take an antacid, take it several hours apart from your calcium/magnesium supplement so you will maximize your mineral uptake. **Calcium channel blockers** prescribed for high blood pressure inhibit the uptake of calcium into the sarcoplasmic reticulum of vascular smooth muscles and cardiac muscles. Since this is likely also true for skeletal muscles, calcium channel blockers would also make trigger points worse, and more difficult to treat. See your health care provider to find out if you can switch to a different medication. Consider treating the underlying causes of hypertension with acupuncture, diet changes, exercise, or whatever is appropriate to your particular set of circumstances.

- **Magnesium deficiency** is less likely to occur as a result of an inadequate dietary intake in a healthy diet as it is to malabsorption, malnutrition, kidney disease, or fluid and electrolyte loss. Magnesium is depleted after strenuous physical exercise, but proper amounts of exercise coupled with an adequate intake of magnesium improves the efficiency of cellular metabolism and improves cardio-respiratory performance. Consumption of alcohol, the use of diuretics, chronic diarrhea, consumption of fluoride, and high amounts of zinc and Vitamin D increase the body's need for magnesium.

  Magnesium is found in most foods, especially dairy products (though this is not recommended for people with damp conditions, such as fibromyalgia), fish, meat, seafood, apples, apricots, avocados, bananas, blackstrap molasses, brewer's yeast, brown rice, figs, garlic, kelp, lima beans, millet, nuts, peaches, black-eyes peas, salmon, sesame seeds, tofu, green leafy vegetable, wheat, and whole grains.

- A diet high in fats, refined sugars, and too much salt causes **potassium deficiency**, as does the use of laxatives and some diuretics. Diarrhea will also deplete potassium. If you suffer from urinary frequency, particularly if your urine is clear rather than light yellow, try taking potassium. Frequent urination causes potassium deficiency, and potassium deficiency may cause frequent urination, and a cycle of depletion ensues. Food sources of potassium include fruit (especially bananas and citrus fruits), potatoes, green leafy vegetables, wheat germ, beans, lentils, nuts, dates, and prunes.

- **Iron deficiency** can lead to **anemia**, and is usually caused by excessive blood loss from a heavy menses, hemorrhoids, intestinal bleeding, donating blood too often, or ulcers. Iron deficiency can also be caused by a long-term illness, prolonged use of antacids, poor digestion, excess coffee or black tea consumption, or the chronic use of NSAID's (non-steroidal anti-inflammatory drugs, such as ibuprofen). Calcium in milk, cheese, or as a supplement can impair absorption of iron, therefore you should take your calcium supplement separately. Do not take an iron supplement if you have an infection or cancer. The body stores it in order to withhold it from bacteria, and in the case of cancer, it may suppress the cancer-killing function of certain cells.

  Early symptoms of iron deficiency include impaired work performance, fatigue, reduced endurance, and an inability to stay warm when exposed to a moderately cold environment. 9-11% of menstruating females in the U.S. are iron deficient, and the world-wide prevalence is about 15%. Iron is best absorbed with Vitamin C. Generally food sources are adequate for improving iron levels for most people. Good sources of iron include eggs, fish, liver, meat, poultry, green leafy vegetables, whole grains, almonds, avocados, beets, blackstrap molasses, brewer's yeast, dates, egg yolks, kelp, kidney and lima beans, lentils, millet, parsley, peaches, pears, dried prunes, pumpkin, raisins, rice and wheat bran, sesame seeds, and soybeans.

One of my favorite books is "*Prescription for Nutritional Healing*" by James F. Balch, M.D., and Phyllis A. Balch, C.N.C.. It has a comprehensive list of vitamins, minerals, amino acids, antioxidants, and enzymes, and food sources for each. It has sections on common disorders listing supplements needed to treat each condition, and helpful hints.

Hormonal Changes

Women are more likely than men to develop trigger points. I have noticed this is particularly true in **menopausal** women. Some teenagers (of both sexes) going through **puberty** also seem to have a tendency to develop trigger points, leading me to believe there is a connection between hormonal changes and one potential cause of trigger points.

Organ Dysfunction and Disease

Thyroid

Both **thyroid inadequacy** (also known as hypometabolism or subclinical hypothyroidism) and **hypothyroidism** will cause and perpetuate trigger points. Hypothyroid patients may experience early morning stiffness, and pain and weakness of the shoulder girdle. Both thyroid inadequacy and hypothyroidism will produce symptoms of cold (and sometimes heat) intolerance, cold hands and feet, muscle aches and pains especially with cold rainy weather, constipation, menstrual problems, weight gain, dry skin, and fatigue and lethargy. Muscles feel rather hard to the touch, and even if a patient is on a thyroid supplement, I've noticed they are still somewhat prone to trigger points, since it is hard to fine-tune the medication exactly to the amount your body would produce if you still had a healthy thyroid organ. Some studies report the prevalence of subclinical hypothyroidism to be as high as 17% in women and 7% in men. Occasionally patients with inadequate metabolism may be thin, nervous, and hyperactive, which may result in a health care provider failing to consider subclinical hypothyroidism.

Patients with low thyroid function may be **low in thiamine (Vitamin B-1)**. Before starting on thyroid medication, try supplementing with thiamine to see if that corrects your thyroid hormone levels. If you are already on thyroid medication and you start taking B-1, you may start exhibiting symptoms of *hyper*thyroidism, and your medication dosage needs to be adjusted. If you are low in B-1 at the time of starting thyroid medication, you may develop symptoms of acute thiamine deficiency, which may be misinterpreted as an intolerance to the medication. After the B-1 deficiency is corrected, you will likely tolerate the medication. You will need to supplement with B-1 prior to and during thyroid hormone therapy to avoid a deficiency. Total body potassium is low in hypothyroidism, and high in hyperthyroidism, so you may need to adjust your potassium intake also.

Smoking impairs the action of thyroid hormone and will make any related symptoms worse. Several pharmaceutical drugs can also affect thyroid hormone levels, such as lithium, anti-convulsants, those that contain iodine, and glucocorticoid steroids, so check with your pharmacist if you have been diagnosed with hypothyroidism and are taking another medication.

A simple **home test** to check your thyroid function is to place a thermometer in your armpit for 10 minutes upon waking but before getting out of bed. Normal underarm temperature for men and post-menopausal women is 98º F (36.7º C). If you are still menstruating your temperature should be around 97.5º F (36.4º C) prior to ovulation, and 98.5º F (36.9º C) following ovulation. If your temperature is lower than this, you will want to check with your health care provider. Often health care providers will only initially **test** the TSH level, which may still be normal if you have hypometabolism rather than hypothyroidism. A radioimmunoassay measures T3 and T4 levels, and gives a more complete picture of the thyroid function.

If you are suffering from depression, be sure to insist that your thyroid levels are tested before starting on anti-depressant medication. I've had more than one patient (especially men) where hypothyroidism was discovered only after they had been medicated for some time.

Hypoglycemia

Both **postprandial (reactive) and fasting hypoglycemia** cause and perpetuate trigger points, and make trigger points more difficult to treat. Symptoms of both are sweating, trembling and shakiness, increased heart rate, and anxiety. Activation of trigger points in the *sternocleidomastoid* muscle by a hypoglycemic reaction may lead to dizziness and headaches. If allowed to progress, symptoms can include visual disturbances, restlessness, and impaired speech and thinking. Missing or delaying a meal does not cause hypoglycemia in a healthy person. A hypoglycemic reaction to a delayed meal usually indicates a problem with the liver, adrenal glands, or pituitary gland. Postprandial hypoglycemia usually occurs two to three hours after eating a meal rich in carbohydrates, and is most like to occur when you are under high stress.

Causes will need to be identified and addressed, if possible. Symptoms will be relieved by eating smaller, more frequent meals with fewer carbohydrates, more protein, and some fat. Avoid all caffeine, alcohol, and tobacco (even second-hand smoke). If you are waking with headaches or pain or having trouble sleeping, try eating a small snack or drink a little juice before bedtime to see if it relieves your symptoms; it usually helps. Acupuncture is quite successful in stabilizing blood sugar.

Gout

Gout will aggravate trigger points and make them difficult to treat. Doctors Travell and Simons recommend keeping the gout under control and taking Vitamin C, and then subsequent treatment of trigger points will be more effective.

Sleep Problems

Pain can interrupt sleep, and interrupted sleep can perpetuate trigger points. It is useful to know whether your sleep was interrupted before your pain started, or whether your sleep was sound and restful. If your sleep was poor prior to the pain, then there is another underlying factor which needs to be addressed to help solve the problem.

Be sure you are not sleeping poorly due to being **too warm or too cold**. If you have

problems falling asleep, try improving your nutrition and your water intake first. Take a calcium/magnesium supplement before bedtime. If you are **waking easily due to noise**, try Mack's™ soft silicon earplugs (my favorite), and try breathing deeply until you fall back to sleep. If you can't stop thinking, you sleep lightly and wake frequently, you wake early and can't fall back to sleep, are menopausal, and/or have vivid and disturbing dreams, try acupuncture and Chinese herbs.

Even if you only drink **caffeine** in the morning, it still disturbs your nighttime sleep pattern, as does **alcohol**. If you choose to give up caffeine, it will take about two weeks before your energy starts to even out and you don't feel like you have to use it to get going in the morning. **Computer use in the evening** stimulates the brain and makes it hard to fall asleep and sleep restfully. If **urinary frequency** is disturbing your sleep, try acupuncture and herbs, and increasing your potassium intake.

Consider whether your **adrenal glands** could be excreting too much cortisol (the "stress hormone"). If you are continually stressed, or if you are pushing yourself too hard and push through fatigue instead of resting or taking a nap, you will excrete more cortisol and have more difficulty sleeping at night. A Naturopathic doctor can administer a saliva test for adrenal function.

Make sure you are not being exposed to **allergens** at night. Get inexpensive soft plastic covers for your pillows and mattress, since many people are allergic to mites, and they live in your bedding. If you have a down comforter or pillow, you may be allergic to the feathers, even if you are not exhibiting classic allergic symptoms, such as sneezing and itchy eyes.

Beds that are too soft can cause a lot of muscular problems, and you may not know it is too soft. Patients usually insist their mattress is firm enough, but when queried further, will admit that sleeping on a mat on the floor gives them relief when the pain is particularly bad. If this is the case, your mattress is not firm enough, no matter how much money you spent on it or how well it worked for someone else. Different people have needs for different kinds of mattresses. An all-cotton futon is very firm, and may be best for some people. The "Sleep Number" bed allows you to change the firmness and some models have an option to control firmness separately for each side of the bed. A lot of people like memory foam beds, but I personally find them too soft. Try putting some camp mats on the floor and sleeping on them for a week. If you feel better, it is time for a new, firmer mattress. Mattresses really only last about five to seven years, and should then be replaced. Some furniture stores will let you try a mattress out for a time period before making a final decision. Be sure you have a **pillow** that keeps your head in line with your spine -- not too high or too low. Sleeping on the couch should definitely be avoided.

If pain disturbs you at night, I sometimes suggest to patients that they keep their self-help ball collection by their bed so that if they wake they can work on their trigger points, and hopefully fall back to sleep once the pain is reduced. The danger in this is that *you have to be sure you don't fall asleep on the ball*! It will cut off the circulation for too long, and make the trigger points worse. It is an easy thing to do when you are fatigued and in pain, and suddenly the pain is reduced or gone, so don't use the ball in bed unless you are sure you will not fall asleep on it.

Spinal Mis-alignments and Other Problems

Vertebrae may be out-of-alignment, and need to be adjusted by a chiropractor or osteopathic physician, or mobilized by a physical therapist. Usually there is also a muscular component that caused the mis-alignment to begin with, so a combined approach of skeletal mobilization and massage or acupuncture is probably necessary for lasting relief. A chiropractor or osteopathic physician will likely take x-rays at the initial visit to evaluate your spine. If you have already had x-rays taken, bring them with you to the visit so you can avoid duplicating x-rays.

Herniated and bulging disks may be very successfully treated with acupuncture (especially Plum Blossom technique), but if you don't get some relief fairly quickly, you may want to consider surgery if you have insurance. Spinal surgery has gotten so sophisticated that many surgeries are fairly minor procedures that have you back on your feet the next day. If you have **stenosis** (a narrowing of the central spinal cord canal or the holes the nerves come out of) acupuncture will help with pain, but not the stenosis, so surgery is probably the best option. With any surgery there is a certain amount of risk, so be sure to discuss this with your operating physician, and make sure you understand the procedure. If you are still unsure, get a second opinion from another surgeon. Disc problems and stenosis need to be confirmed with an MRI.

Bone spurs and narrowed disc spaces can cause pain. But in a random sample of the population you will find many people with bone spurs and narrowed disc spaces with no pain, and many people with pain and no bone spurs or narrowed disc spaces, so don't assume these are causing your problems, even if a health care provider has made this assumption.

I always start with the assumption that trigger points are at least part of the problem, if not all of the problem, and treat accordingly. If a patient doesn't receive some relief fairly quickly, then I know there may be something else going on and I refer them to someone who can evaluate them with an x-ray or MRI.

If you have had surgery and your pain continues, trigger points are the likely culprit, and need to be treated for lasting relief. If you still do not get relief, there is a possibility the pain is due to scar tissue from the surgery compressing a nerve root, so you will need to check with your health care provider.

Laboratory Tests

Laboratory tests may be necessary to help diagnose some of the systemic perpetuating factors. With blood chemistry profiles, an elevated erythrocyte sedimentation rate (**SED Rate**) may indicate a chronic bacterial infection, polymyositis, polymyalgia rheumatica, rheumatoid arthritis, or cancer. A decreased **erythrocyte count** and/or **low hemoglobin** points to anemia. A mean corpuscular volume (**MCV**) of over 92fl indicates the likelihood of a folate or B-12 deficiency. **Eosinophilia** may indicate an allergy or intestinal parasitic infection. An increase in **monocytes** can indicate low thyroid function, infectious mononucleosis, or an acute viral infection. Increased serum **cholesterol** can be caused by a problem with low thyroid function, and a low serum cholesterol can indicate folate deficiency. High **uric acid** levels indicate hyperuricemia and possibly gout.

Iron deficiency is detected by checking the **serum ferritin** level. A **fasting blood test** is used to diagnose hypoglycemia, and an additional **glucose tolerance test** or a 2-hour postprandial blood glucose test may be used to rule out diabetes. (Measurement of **sensory**

nerve conduction velocities can help diagnose diabetic neuropathy.) A low serum total calcium suggests a calcium deficiency, but for an accurate assessment of the available calcium, a **serum ionized calcium** test needs to be performed. **Potassium** levels can be checked with a serum potassium test.

Blood tests can determine **serum levels of Vitamins B-1, B-6, B-12, folic acid, and Vitamins C and D.** Any values in the lower 25% of the normal range or below would indicate that supplementation would be helpful in the treatment of trigger points. Remember that even if serum levels of vitamins and minerals are normal, you may still wish to use supplements since tissue supplies will drop before the body allows serum levels in the blood to drop.

See the above section on Nutritional Problems for comments on the digestive system and vitamin and mineral sources. See the above section on Organ Dysfunction and Disease for a discussion of thyroid function tests. A hair analysis can detect high levels of toxic metals exposure and deficiencies in minerals. A naturopathic doctor can perform **blood tests for food allergies**. Stool samples will reveal if **parasites** are a problem.

APPENDIX B

What Are Trigger Points?

Muscle Anatomy & Physiology

Muscles consist of many muscle cells, or *fibers* bundled together by connective tissue. Each fiber contains numerous *myofibrils*, and most skeletal muscles contain approximately one thousand to two thousand myofibrils. Each myofibril consists of a chain of *sarcomeres* connected end-to-end. Muscular contractions take place in the sarcomere.

A *muscle spindle* is a sensory receptor found within the belly of a muscle. Muscle spindles are concentrated where a nerve enters a muscle, and around nerves inside the muscles. Each spindle is composed of three to twelve *intrafusal muscle fibers*, which detect changes in the length of a muscle. As the body's position changes, information is conveyed to the central nervous system via sensory neurons, and is processed in the brain. As needed, the *motor end plate* (a type of nerve ending) releases *acetylcholine*, a neurotransmitter that tells the *sarcoplasmic reticulum* (part of each cell) to release ionized calcium. The *extrafusal muscle fibers* then contract. When contraction of the muscle fibers are no longer needed, the nerve ending stops releasing acetylcholine and the calcium pump within the sarcoplasmic reticulum re-uptakes calcium.

Trigger Point Physiology: Contractions and Inflammation

One of the current theories about the mechanism responsible for the formation of trigger points is the "Integrated Trigger Point Hypothesis." If a trauma occurs or there is a large increase in the motor end plate's release of acetylcholine, an excessive amount of calcium can be released by the sarcoplasmic reticulum. This causes a maximal contracture of a segment of muscle, leading to a maximal demand for energy and impairment of local circulation. If circulation is impaired, the calcium pump doesn't get the fuel and oxygen it needs to pump calcium back into the sarcoplasmic reticulum, so the muscle fiber stays contracted. Sensitizing substances are released, causing pain and stimulation of the autonomic nervous system, resulting in a positive feedback system with the motor nerve terminal releasing excessive acetylcholine...and so the sarcomere stays contracted.

Another current theory is the "Muscle Spindle" hypothesis, which proposes that the main cause of a trigger point is an inflamed muscle spindle (Partanen, Ojala, and Arokoski, 2010). Pain receptors activate skeletofusimotor units during sustained overload of muscles via a spinal reflex pathway which connect to the muscle spindles. As pain continues, sustained contraction and fatigue drive the skeletofusimotor units to exhaustion, and cause rigor (silent spasm) of the extrafusal muscle fibers, forming the "taut band" we feel as trigger points. Because the muscle spindle itself has a poor blood supply, the contraction and inflammatory metabolites released will be concentrated inside the spindle and lead to sustained inflammation.

A ground-breaking 2008 study (Shah et al.) was able to measure eleven elevated biochemicals in and surrounding active trigger points, including inflammatory mediators, neuropeptides, catecholamines, and cytokines (primarily sensitizing substances and immune system biochemicals). In addition, the pH of the samples was strongly acidic compared to other areas of the body. A 1996 study by Issbener, Reeh, and Steen found that a localized acidic pH lowers the pain threshold sensitivity level of sensory receptors (part of the nervous system), even without acute damage to the muscle. This means the more acidic your pH level in a given area, the more easily you will experience pain compared to someone else. Further studies are needed to discover whether body-wide elevations in pH acidity and the substances mentioned above predispose people to develop trigger points.

More studies are needed to determine the exact mechanisms of trigger point formation and physiology.

Central Sensitization, Trigger Points, and Chronic Pain

The *autonomic nervous system* controls the release of acetylcholine, along with involuntary functions of blood vessels and glands. Anxiety and nervous tension increase autonomic nervous system activity, which commonly aggravates trigger points and their associated symptoms.

The *central nervous system* includes the brain and spinal cord, and its function is to integrate and coordinate all activities and responses of the body. The purpose of the *acute* stress responses of our bodies is to protect us by telling us to pull away from a hot stove burner, flee from a dangerous situation, or rest an injured body part due to pain. But when emotional or physical stress is prolonged, even just for days, there is a maladaptive response: damage to the central nervous system, particularly to the sympathetic nervous system and the hypothalamus-pituitary-adrenal (HPA) systems. This is called *central nervous system sensitization.*

Pain causes certain types of nerve receptors in muscles to relay information to *neurons* located within part of the gray matter of the spinal cord and the brain stem. Pain is amplified there and then is relayed to other muscles, thereby expanding the region of pain beyond the initially affected area. Persistent pain leads to long-term or possibly permanent changes in these neurons, which affect adjacent neurons through *neurotransmitters.*

Various substances are released: *histamine* (a compound that causes dilation and permeability of blood vessels), *serotonin* (a neurotransmitter that constricts blood vessels), *bradykinin* (a hormone that dilates peripheral blood vessels and increases small blood vessel permeability), and *substance P* (a compound involved in the regulation of the pain threshold). These substances stimulate the nervous system to release even more acetylcholine locally, adding to the perpetuation of trigger points.

Central sensitization may cause the part of the nervous system that would normally counteract pain to malfunction and fail to do its job. As a result, pain can both be more easily triggered by lower levels of physical and emotional stressors, and also be more intense and last longer. Prolonged pain caused by central nervous system sensitization can lead to emotional and physical stress. Conversely, prolonged exposure to both emotional and physical stressors can lead to central nervous system sensitization and subsequently cause pain. Just the central nervous system maladaptive changes alone can be self-perpetuating and cause pain, even without the presence of either the original or any additional stressors, creating a vicious cycle of pain and trigger point formation.

Once the central nervous system is involved, because of central sensitization, even if the original perpetuating factor causing trigger points are resolved, trigger points can continue being formed and reactivated. So the longer pain goes untreated, the greater the number of neurons that get involved and the more muscles they affect, causing pain in new areas, in turn causing more neurons to get involved…the bigger the problem becomes, leading to the likelihood that pain will become chronic. The problem gets more complex, more painful, more debilitating, more frustrating, and more time-consuming and expensive to treat. The longer you wait, the less likely you are to get complete relief, and the more likely it is that your trigger points will be reactivated chronically and periodically. The sooner pain is treated, including addressing the initiating stressors and perpetuating factors, the less likely it will become a permanent problem with widespread muscle involvement and central nervous system changes.

How Will You Know if You Have Trigger Points?

The two most important characteristics of trigger points that you will notice are tender knots or tight bands in the muscles, and referred pain. You may also notice weakness, lack of range-of-motion, or other symptoms you would not normally associate with muscular problems.

Tenderness, "Knots," and Tight Bands in the Muscle

When pressed, trigger points are usually very tender. This is because the sustained contraction of the myofibril leads to the release of sensitizing neurotransmitters via a cascade effect: the sustained contraction elevates metabolites such as potassium ions and lactic acid, which leads to the elevated levels of inflammatory agents such as bradykinin and histamine, which activates pain nerve fibers, which leads to the excretion of pain transmitters, such as substance P.

Pain intensity levels can vary depending on the amount of stress placed on the muscles. The intensity of pain can also vary in response to flare-ups of any of the perpetuating factors addressed in Appendix A, and the presence of central sensitization (see above). The areas at the ends of the muscle fibers also become tender, either at the bone or where the muscle attaches to a tendon.

Healthy muscles usually do not contain knots or tight bands, are not tender to pressure, and, when not in use, feel soft and pliable to the touch, not like the hard and dense muscles found in people with chronic pain. People often tell me their muscles feel hard and dense because they work out and do strengthening exercises, but healthy muscles feel soft and pliable when not being used, even if you work out. Muscles with trigger points may also be relaxed, so don't assume you do not have trigger points just because the muscle is *not* hard and dense.

Referred Pain

Trigger points may refer pain both in the area in which the trigger point is located, and/or to other areas of the body. These are called *referral patterns*. About half of commonly found trigger points are not located within their area of referred pain. The most common referral patterns have been well documented and diagramed, and are found in the muscle chapters in section III of this book.

Unless you know where to search for trigger points, and you only work on the areas where you feel pain, you probably won't get relief. For example, trigger points in the iliopsoas muscle (deep in your abdomen) can cause pain in your lumbar area. If you don't check the iliopsoas muscle for trigger points, and only work on the quadratus lumborum muscle in the lumbar area, you will not get relief.

There are approximately four hundred muscles in the human body, but a few muscles may or may not be present in some people. Any muscle can develop trigger points, potentially causing referred pain and other symptoms. There are also individual variations in fiber or tendon arrangement, so trigger points may be located in different places for different people.

Weakness and Muscle Fatigue

Trigger points can cause weakness and loss of coordination, along with an inability to use the muscle. Many people take this as a sign that they need to strengthen the weak muscles, but you can't condition (strengthen) a muscle that contains trigger points -- these muscle fibers are not available for use because they are already contracted. If trigger points aren't inactivated first, strengthening (*conditioning*) exercises will likely encourage the surrounding muscles to do the work instead of the muscle containing the trigger point, further weakening and deconditioning the muscle containing trigger points.

Muscles containing trigger points are fatigued more easily and don't return to a relaxed state as quickly when you stop using the muscle. Trigger points may cause other muscles to tighten up and become weak and fatigued in the areas where you experience the referred pain, and also cause a generalized tightening of an area as a response to pain.

Other Symptoms

Trigger points can cause symptoms that most people would not normally associate with muscular problems. For example, trigger points in the abdominal muscles can cause urinary frequency and bladder spasms, bed-wetting, chronic diarrhea, frequent belching and gas, nausea, loss of appetite, heartburn, food intolerance, painful menses, projectile vomiting, testicular pain, and pain that feels like it is in an organ, in addition to causing referred pain in the abdominal, mid-back, and lumbar areas.

Trigger points may also cause stiff joints, generalized weakness or fatigue, twitching, trembling, and areas of numbness or other odd sensations. It probably wouldn't occur to you (or your health care provider) that these symptoms could be caused by a trigger point in a muscle.

Sensitization of the Opposite Side of the Body

For any long-term pain, it's not unusual for both sides of the body to eventually be affected; for example, if the right lumbar area is painful, there may be tender points in the left lumbar area. Often the opposite side is actually *more* tender with pressure. This is because whatever is affecting one side is likely affecting the other: poor body mechanics, poor footwear, overuse injuries, chronic degenerative or inflammatory conditions, chronic disease, or central sensitization. For that reason, I almost always treat both sides on patients, and I recommend that you do self-treatments on both sides. You may find that you have trigger points only on one side for any given muscle, but always check both sides before making that assumption.

Active Trigger Points vs. Latent Trigger Points

If a trigger point is *active*, it will refer pain or other sensations and limit range of motion. If a trigger point is *latent*, it may cause a decreased range of motion and weakness, but not pain. The more frequent and intense your pain, the greater the number of active trigger points you likely have.

Trigger points that start with some impact to the muscle, such as an injury, are usually active initially. Poor posture or poor body mechanics, repetitive use, a nerve root irritation, or any of the other perpetuating factors addressed in Appendix A can also form active trigger points. Latent trigger points can develop gradually without being active first, and you don't even know they are there. Most people have at least some latent trigger points, which can easily be converted to active trigger points.

Active trigger points may at some point stop referring pain and become latent. However, these latent trigger points can easily become active again, which may lead you to believe you're experiencing a new problem when in fact an old problem—perhaps even something you've forgotten about—is being reaggravated. Any of the perpetuating factors discussed in Appendix A can activate previously latent trigger points and make you more prone to developing new trigger points initiated by impacts to muscles.

What Initiates and Perpetuates Trigger Points?

Trigger points may form after a sudden trauma or injury, or they may develop gradually. Common initiating and perpetuating factors are mechanical stresses, injuries, nutritional problems, emotional factors, sleep problems, acute or chronic infections, organ dysfunction and disease, and other medical conditions.

You will have more control over some perpetuating factors than others. Addressing any pertinent perpetuating factors is so important that you may obtain either a great amount or complete relief from pain without any additional treatment. If you don't eliminate perpetuating factors to the extent possible, you may not get more than temporary relief from self-help pressure techniques or practitioners' treatments. Hopefully, you will learn enough about the perpetuating factors in Appendix A that at least if you choose not to resolve them, you are making an informed choice about whether the relief of pain is more important to you than continuing to do things that make you feel worse.

You cannot realistically make all of the changes in the muscle chapters and Appendix A all at once, but make a list of the perpetuating factors that might apply to you. Prioritize and work on resolving those you think might be most important.

Other Books by the Author

Pain Relief with Trigger Point Self Help, DeLaune, Valerie LAc

Flashdrive format (2004, revised 2012, 2017). A multimedia book-on-Flashdrive for pain relief, appropriate for both practitioners and the lay public. It contains information on the causes and locations of trigger points for the entire body, along with hundreds of color photos with overlays of common pain referral patterns, and 144 video clips of self-help techniques for applying pressure to trigger points and performing stretches. A search feature allows you to search for your related medical conditions. Because the book navigates in your web browser, it is easy to locate the source of your pain, and move from one relevant chapter to the next.

It contains introductory chapters on the physiology and characteristics of trigger points, and a comprehensive chapter on all of the perpetuating factors that can cause and keep trigger points activated, along with solutions. Perpetuating factors include poor ergonomics and poorly-designed furniture, clothing problems, inadequate nutrition, inadequate water, improper diet, injuries, spinal and skeletal factors, sleep problems, emotional factors, allergies, hormonal imbalances, organ dysfunction or disease, and acute or chronic viral, bacterial, or parasitic infections. For more information on how to purchase this book, and for additional resources, go to http://triggerpointrelief.com/

Other Titles by Valerie DeLaune, LAc

Trigger Point Therapy Workbook for Upper Back and Neck Pain (2nd ed., 2013) Anchorage: Institute of Trigger Point Studies (e-pub, Print-on-Demand)

Trigger Point Therapy Workbook for Shoulder Pain including Frozen Shoulder (2nd ed., 2013) Anchorage: Institute of Trigger Point Studies (e-pub, Print-on-Demand)

Trigger Point Therapy Workbook for Lower Back and Gluteal Pain (2nd ed., 2013) Anchorage: Institute of Trigger Point Studies (e-pub, Print-on-Demand)

Trigger Point Therapy Workbook for Chest and Abdominal Pain (2013) Anchorage: Institute of Trigger Point Studies (e-pub)

Trigger Point Therapy Workbook for Headaches & Migraines including TMJ Pain (2013) Anchorage: Institute of Trigger Point Studies (e-pub)

Trigger Point Therapy Workbook for Lower Arm Pain including Elbow, Wrist, Hand & Finger Pain (2013) Anchorage: Institute of Trigger Point Studies (e-pub)

Trigger Point Therapy Workbook for Knee, Leg, Ankle, and Foot Pain (2018) Anchorage: Institute of Trigger Point Studies (e-pub, Print-on-Demand)

For more information on how to purchase these books, and for additional resources, go to http://triggerpointrelief.com/

"Like" the *author* on Facebook at Facebook.com: Valerie-DeLaune

"Like" the *Institute of Trigger Point Studies* on Facebook at Facebook.com: Institute-of-Trigger-Point-Studies